W9-AUJ-961

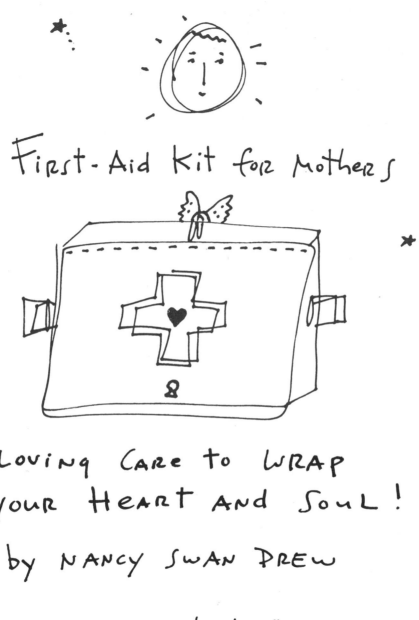

First-Aid Kit for Mothers

Loving Care to WRAP your HEART AND SouL!

by NANCY SWAN DREW

* Celestial Arts

Berkeley / Toronto

Celestial Arts
P.O. Box 7123
Berkeley, California 94707

A Heart + Star Book

Library of Congress Cataloging-in-
Publication Data

Drew, Nancy Swan
   First-Aid kit for Mothers: Loving
      Care to wrap your Heart and
      Soul!/by Nancy Swan Drew
      p. cm.
   ISBN 0-89087-861-7 (paper)
   1. Obstetrics-- Miscellanea. 2. Motherhood--
      Miscellanea. I. Title.
   RG121 . D775 2000
   618.2 -- dc21   99-056534

First printing, 2000
12345 - 04 03 02 01 00

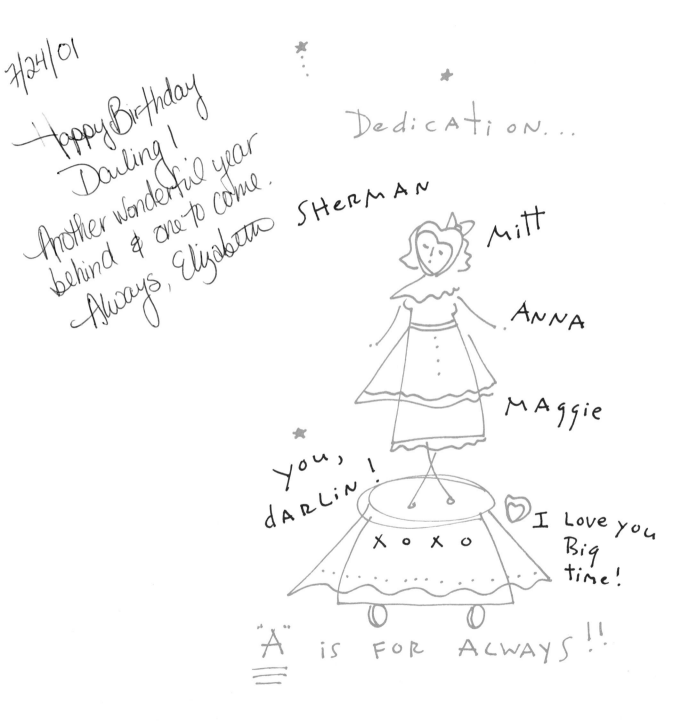

7/24/01

Happy Birthday Darling! Another wonderful year behind & one to come. Always, Elizabeth

Dedication...

SHERMAN

Mitt

ANNA

MAGGIE

you, DARLIN!

XOXO

I Love you Big time!

"A" is FOR ALWAYS!!

Table of Contents

*..

Introduction

Dear Sweet Reader _____!

By the time I was in the fourth grade at St. Hugo's, it was clear to me that I would someday become an artist. I felt this to be true because when I was coloring, cutting, and pasting I felt WHOLE.

No three-layer cake, Saturday
morning cartoon, or sneaky venial
sin could give me that glorious
feeling. I loved it so much I
worked to know it again and
again.

No

yes

Along the way to grown-
up land there have been other

experiences, mighty fine indeed, that have added to my "whole" picture. Falling in love, loving best friends, discovering the silken threads of understanding that gift wrap families, and engaging, through nature, in daily chit-chats with the master artist of all BEAUTY.

My better-than-best lotto ticket in the winning of completeness came my way when I became what many of us are... A mother. This "job"... "calling"... "role"... that defines you and me, is a great mystery to be solved in little sturdy steps.

Like playing in a championship,
there are seasons of bliss and
others that salute the loyal
will of the Chicago Cubs.

This book is a personal
map and gift to your mothering
HEARt. It is a trophy to
sit atop your nightstand for
All that you do and are... trips

x

to the E.R. , school playground,
grocery store ... the hours of
dawn, greeted alone, as you
worry a new day awake.
Your sometimes "too tired to
think" life has more merit
and unclaimed distinction than
a million steps on the moon or
pirated jewels that (no matter

xi

how lovely...) fail to buy your dreams come true. This job, darlin, is A high HIGH

HONOR.

Sadly, the Face of the world hAS yet to bestow upon mother-hood ♥ its proper grace And gratitude. In time... your own children will <u>see</u> this "CALLING" for what it is: the noble art of loving someone into full bloom. I really think that a slice of heaven on earth is found in the children who have been mothered by champions, like you. Your Oscars are your children, the bouquets you gather and leave behind.

Love,
Nancy Drew

xiii

P.S. There is no Microwavable recipe for perfect mothering... It is an hourly mix that melts into years of stepping up to bat... Don't be afraid... Say, "give me the ball, little darlin... I can do this... give me the ball." Whether a single mom, or married to a swell guy, a career-gal mom, stay-

At-home mom, Foster mom, grandmère, or cooler-than-cool-aunt... No matter how you chop up the parts of your life to create your own remarkable recipe, ALWAYS REMEMBER: for one part DISCIPLINE, Add TEN parts LOVE; for one part wisdom, Add ten parts LOVE... And so it goes, dolly.

XV

Stir and mix... sit and watch...
softly pray and, lo and behold,
your very own GOLDEN
mothering STEW... so complete
and true.

xvi

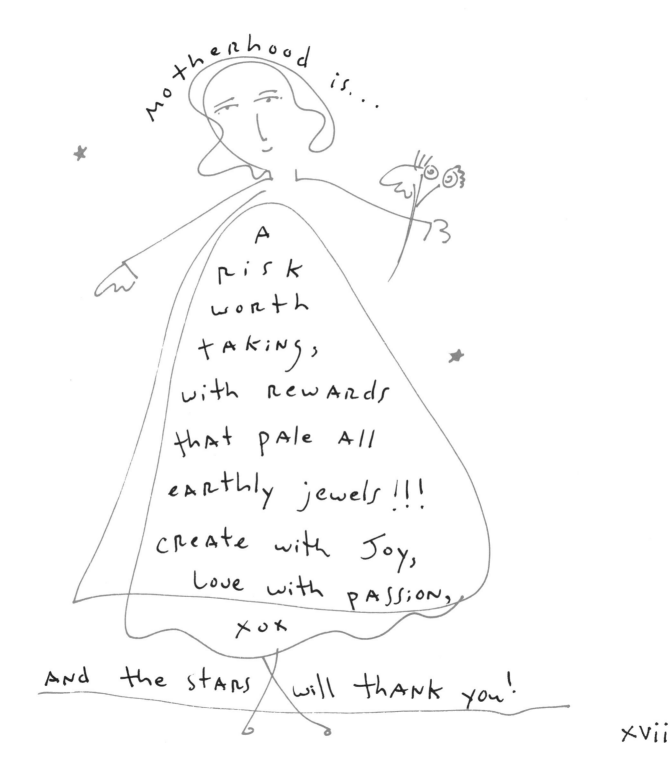

motherhood is...

A risk worth taking, with rewards that pale all earthly jewels!!! create with Joy, love with passion, xox

and the stars will thank you!

xvii

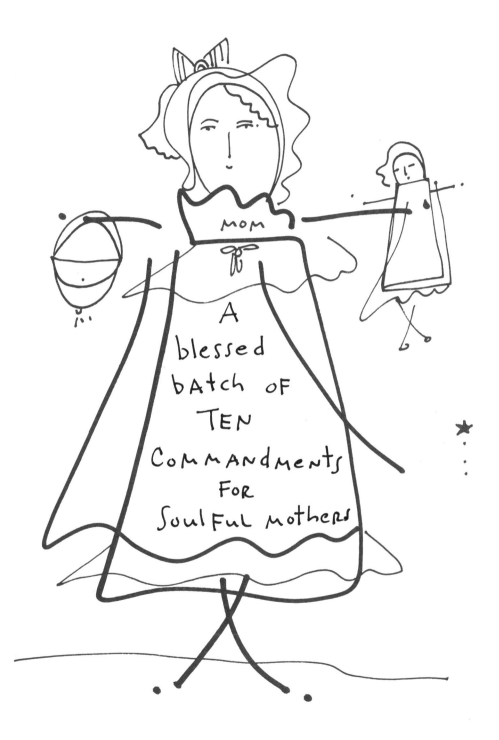

MOM

A
blessed
bAtch oF
TEN
CommANdments
FoR
SoulFul mothers

I. I shall not own all that is good or bad within my children's universe.

II. No matter what... I shall NEVER EVER GIVE UP !!!

III. I shall not allow mistakes to derail my MATERNAL locomotive...

Bumps

MOM

Kids

WHOA... "I think I can... I know I can!!!

xix

IV. I shall Forgive my parents ASAP for whatever "change" I was shorted that may or may not have ever existed in their emotional piggy bank.

V. I shall regard my private museum of Broken Hearts as a mighty collection of "Purple Hearts" for high courage and loving nobility. [trophy Room] P.S. Change your specs!

xx

VI. I shall embrace each day of mothering, knowing that ALL children are MIRACLES ON LOAN, AND I AM one Lucky Duck!!!

VII. I shall, when wrong, apologize to my children and try with all my heart to better my mistakes. False pride is a wicked Hobby.

VIII. I shall applaud my victories and be ever so grateful for all in love that holds us near and tight.

xxi

<u>IX</u>. I shall not be blue and rattled <u>IF</u> I do not look exactly like I did on my wedding day... "Mirror Mirror on the wall... show me my INNER BEAUTY... AFTER ALL!"

★ ★

<u>X</u>. I shall MEASURE my words like a fine chef, careful to follow the expert mix of delicate ingredients in a mother's BEST recipe: "LUV-PIE"!

P.S. Button ANGRY lips, darlin'!

XOX

CHAPTER I.

BAMBINO DAZE...
PREGNANCY...

Well dolly, this short and seemingly never-ending blink of time is much like carrying a secret renter just beneath your heart. Imagine yourself... as a tall castle and in your innermost corridor is a prince or princess (or both) awaiting their debut. This wondrous arrangement may give you

1.

the following sensations:

☆ Flying to the moon and back, lickety-split.

☆ Fear... worry... puzzlement!!

☆ An upset tummy, as though you had just gone on the most virtually horrific ride at the fair, after a five-course supper.

☆ Joy... more than your best holidays... in one batch... tripled twice!

☆ A sense of completeness that one often spends a lifetime wanting and needing.

2.

☆ your blue days may give you a fantasy of working part-time at the nearest circus as the "Robust Madonna in waiting." xox

☆ your platinum days, however, will take your weary spirits to a high throne: motherhood, darlin!!!

Every time I spot a woman with child... on the street or in a crowd, I have a brief rush of happiness for MYSELF and my memory bank. Such a courageous job she has... THIS high honor, mother-child partnership, that begins with a blind love, that like a magic carpet, will take them anywhere they wish to go. Up... down... all around clouds of rain and stars that promise

4.

to shine well past the ink-black night.

In my own experience, I preferred the times of "womb Aerobics"... when clearly my little one was Rockin' and Rollin' to its own Abstract tunes. With each nudge and kick I fell in love with this baby... deeper and

D e e p e r.

yes, I did.

THE future, darlin, may bring a different series of nudges and kicks that mightily tests your Mettle. This... is why it is one dandy miracle to revisit your "Bambino Daze", perhaps to draw upon an invisible bank account that is called "Eternal Love... No Matter What", opened the very moment your secret renter arrived inside your castle... just beneath your Heart.

6.

Dottie loved being pregnant... It made her feel worthwhile.

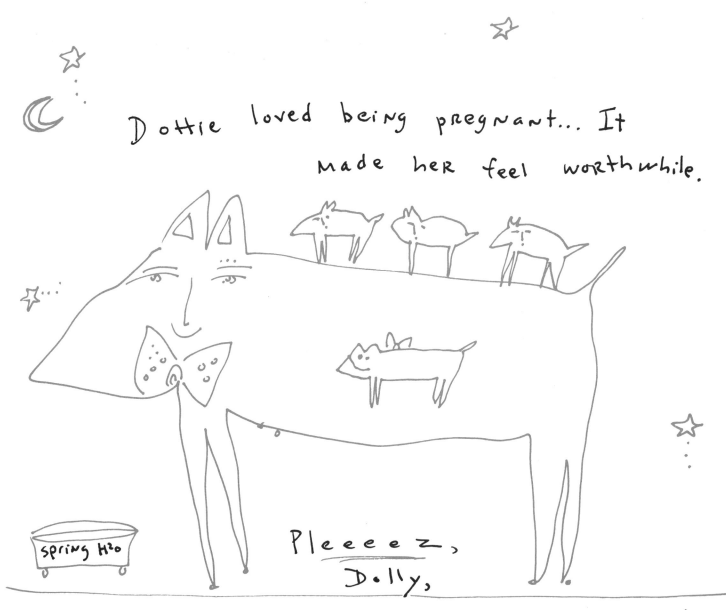

spring H2O

Pleeeez, Dolly,

DeFine yourSelF AS exceptionally worthwhile well before you commit to this "career."

7.

SECRET.....PERSONAL MOMENTS OF MINE... *1970's*

☆ Having A strong Reliance on salted

cashews And chocolate malts thick enough

to be porridge.   souPY gooP... tsk tsk!!!

☆ Despising support hose in putty- tan

colors... mid-August!! Hating sack dresses,
    better suited For soFA upholstery.

☆ Really not liking the uninvited stories

from strangers And Faux friends about

the very worst things that could possibly

8. happen, TRue or False, as they might be.

☆ Beginning Nice projects (domestic cleaning) And Running out of FUEL to complete them At day's end. Very weary, indeed. (This is A Huge clue to dAys Ahead.)

☆ Waiting in the Doctor's office... Will that ever chAnge??? Will the Doctor ever be early or give "bonus coupons" to A massage therApist, For every moment of WAiting??

LAte...
AgaiN...

Next!!

NuRse

Doctor

GEEEZ...

☆ And... could their reading material be elevated?!? If you were not nervous before you arrived... don't read any-thing... Bring your own or learn to knit.

☆ BATTLING Seat belts that couldn't reach without a tug-of-war!!

☆ Ignoring Relatives who said, "Don't buy A thing for the nursery, etc., until right before theee delivery... just in case something goes wrong... don't you know?!?

10.

Listening to student nurses in the waiting room, discussing, over my mile-high womb, what brand of used appliances to buy for their boyfriends' birthdays. I'm amazed that they could keep Track of my contractions and select an avocado-green range at the same time.

Experiencing full labor and then a bonus: the unexpected C-section. This workout would have been Jane Fonda's nightmare...without a cute spandex zorro suit.

11.

✳ My very first outing, After the birth of my son was to every mom's favorite spot... the local pharmacy. A sweet woman asked me how my son was doing... "you know, darlin... the lawyer". Well she meant my husband, of course. I walked straight to the beauty creams and bought two of each.

✳ Holding my baby for the very first time... gave the word GIFT a supernatural Halo.

12.

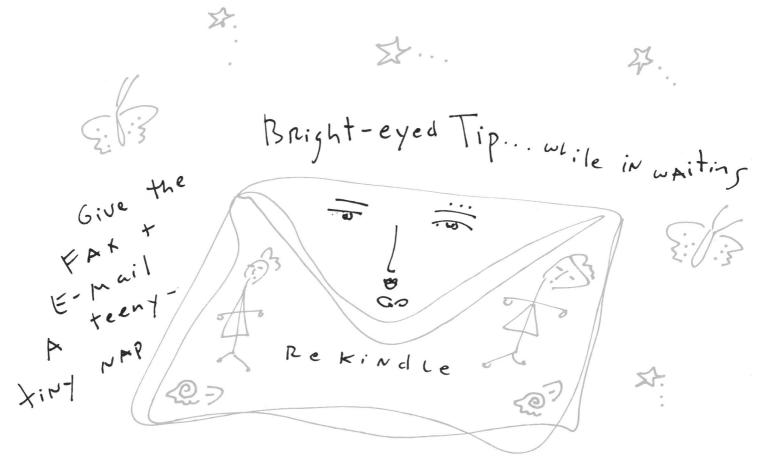

Bright-eyed Tip... while in waiting

Give the FAX + E-mail A teeny-tiny NAP

Rekindle

Discover AN old mode of civilized connections: A gift of thought, Time, And the HAND's Heart-driven pulse. Script AN original LETTER to A pAL.. one true love.. etc. on Lovely papers with your illustrations!!!

13.

Ready your nest... A S A P...
Bit by Bit...

Set realistic GOALS... Pitch... Purge...
Make-do... Redo... get A brand-
new HAiRdo... All of those tasks
that Healthy lists Are made of...
March FORWARD At a steady clip!!

OH such mmm...
RECOGNiZAble
Results...
my gosh...

this can be
GREAT
FUN...

14.

Darlin Love...

☆ Lists can be grounding maps and perpetual monitors of moving forward.

Now.. FOR YOU ..As a grown-up mother-to-be...

I do advocate the art and high power of list making. This can only hurt if you are under the horrid spell that all lists must be completed by sundown. If this is your natural disposition, ignore this First-Aid Band-Aid and cover more open Prairies with your wealthy therapist. As for the rest of us we will rejoice in the "Checking Off" ☑ of one more thing... 15.

keep a revolving... evolving...

Begin At the top... Move down-ward... or bounce All About !!!
if you so Fanceee...

☆ CLOSETS.... BASEMENT.... Attic!!

☆ PLACES WHERE you store And hide!! FACE this challenge At your highest energy crest. work to music that nudges you swiftly toward decision making. IDENtiFy your "things" by writing info on boxes. If you hate to part company... be brAve, give A batch to Goodwill !!

purr-fect!

BAH-Bye!

xoxox

1b.

THE kitchen... This really is the heart of your nest. Pretend you are a master surgeon, called upon daily to perform life-affirming acts of brilliance. See your post-pregnant self suiting up in new blue jeans and checkered aprons, gathering formula and sterilizing bottles. Just imagine those happy days... with a streamlined spic-and-span operating kitchen!

Ready to go... doll!

17.

- ☐ ♡   Pitch old Rusted gAdgets. Go to the "dollAR" OR "zillion" dollAR store + voilA!!   New   Fresh

- ☐ ♡   Buy extRA - FResh, blue and white towels And dish cloths !!! splurge!

- ☐ ♡   Check your condiments + staples. Buy two of your Favorites to get you through quick Hops to the 7-Eleven. TRy to Avoid excessive eRRAND RunNing. When the BAMBiNo ARRives, you would much RAtheR "cuddle" thAn scoot about.

1♂.

- ☐ ♡ Clean windows and curtains. Line shelves, drawers...clean baseboards, windowsills. APPLIANCES TOO!!

- ☐ ♡ Map out baby equipment... infant Feeding chair (safe), high chair!!

    *Serious Home Camping Tips!

- ☐ ♡ Buy Extra: toilet paper, paper towels, NAPKINS, dishwasher soap, trash bags, light bulbs, pet food, Tylenol, toothpaste, deodorant, laundry soap. Pretend you are going on an extended trip within your own home. Return to normal date... unknown!!

Sleeping Quarters

☐ ♡   Soften... brighten... Freshen up the rooms that offer quiet sanctuary. Discover what hides beneath the bed, Delete the unnecessary, Line drawers with sweet-scented papers. Arrange framed photos of all your favorite people (include some relatives... dolly!). Scatter clothbound books of substance for those pokey days when your little darlin is a-napping and the clock is kind.

When life is in a transition, and gears shift... Embrace the adventure with visual reminders of tried-and-true comforts! Photos of family and pals... this is oh so helpful, especially if you've moved miles from what your interior map calls "home". Build a MAZE of clear Kodak mementos and save your dough-re-me for the phone bill!!!

21.

- ☐ ♡ The Royal Nursery... In a way, this <u>is</u> a gift to the preparer... because the bambino will be far too busy growing in the first months to even applaud the decorating. So darlin, delight your fairy-tale whims and play away with color and pattern, fuzzy teddy bears and moonbeam wishes, remember a trusty <u>rocking chair!!!</u>

22. ☆ Gosh, is your comfy nest finished ▱ ??

Master List cont.

- ☐ ♡ Bathrooms and laundry stations... Equip them with backup goods. (Purchase anti-bacterial products) Stock for your sweet self notions that will pamper you for the bath!! Lavender will calm you, Gardenia will surprise you, Sooo... in a secret spot, stash private luxuries, including mini-books to explore while in the tub!! Be sure to put the rubber duckie out-of-sight when you have a SPA-moment.

Write your soon-to-be little one
a love letter full of your high
dreams and landscapes of hope.
Take lots of time with this... seal
it with a kiss and hide it away, until
your child's turn in the road
tells you it is time, time to
open this first scripting of a
mother's heart.

For... Susan
Love Mom
date

24.

Bright-Eyed Tip

NEST-PREP

SOLO EFFORTS?? MMM...

TEAMWORK is best when there is a sharp delegater. Perhaps all of your tasks will be "cooperative" efforts, with the help of a pal, sister or mate... Or hire a FAB future baby-sitter to give you a hand!! Take this time to interview well !.!.!.

25.

BRAVO... DARLIN, YOUR NEST IS ALL Perky And Bright, And your little one's debut is ONLY A Few heart-beats AWAy. LiFe's wheel is declaring ⎯ I pray that of Fortune yours to be even-so Brilliant!!!

P.S. When At the hospital, if you do find physical discomfort A distraction, Aunt Pearl suggests you speak up and Ask the Doctor for some MEDS! Focus back onto the grand event!!!

First-Aid

Band-Aids for Bambino Daze...

Apply as needed, little darlin...

s.o.s.

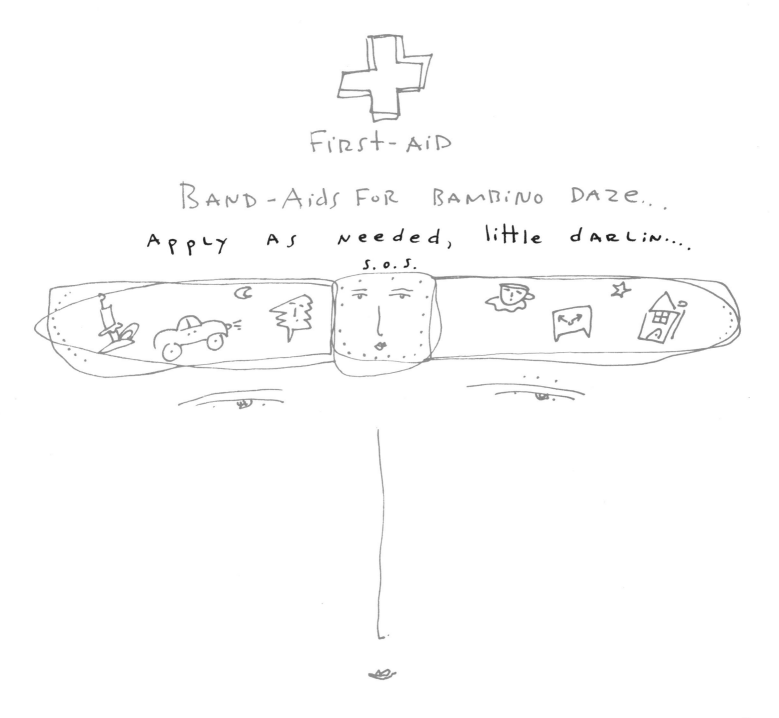

First - Aid
For BAMBINO... DAZE...

TREAT YOURSELF to A BOUNTY OF
Sweet DREAMS... SLEEP, DARLIN... TAKE
petite MADONNA NAPS AS you wish!!
You ARE the ARCHITECT OF A BRAND-
NEW Life within... Rest FOR TWO!!

Feed your guest a feast of good things: Fruits and vegetables from the garden of great expectations. Prepare them well and present them on royal servers. Take the time to fuss over your "fuel" agenda. Drive-thrus, darlin, do not befit a Queen-in-waiting...

Use your best china and crystal...Who on earth are you waiting for... Elvis?

H₂O

29.

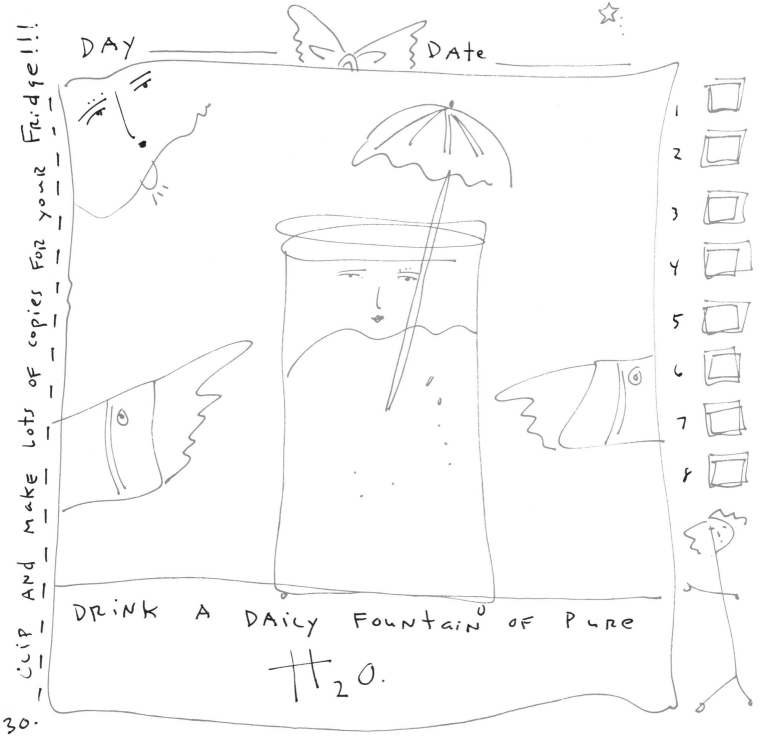

DAY _____   DATE _____

Clip and make lots of copies for your Fridge!!!

DRINK A DAILY FOUNTAIN OF PURE H_2O.

1
2
3
4
5
6
7
8

30.

A mother's BANQUET GiFts to
CHild

BREAKFAST...

LUNCH ....

SUPPER ....

SNACKS... Kind oNes with A purpose...

31.

sweet wishes

☆ SELECT NINE things you wish to
DO FOR YOURSELF before the big
Birthday. PLAN it AS A monthly
Road Marker!!! e.g. A mini-trip. Visit
with A pal... Museum... spA-day...

1.
2.
3.
4.
5.
6.
7.
8.
9.

GOOD IDEA... DARLIN... ☾

CREATE A separate Log or Journal
FOR your daily or weekly or hit-and-
miss feelings And mindful snippets.
PLACE AN old baby photo of your
sweet SELF (A baby picture of the Father, if
you so wish) on the cover And Leave
the very LAST page for A first photo
of theee BAMBINO!! SomedAy, long
from now, shARe this with your son
or daughter. It will bind you in
Another grAnd way. PerhAps title it
"MY GREAT ExpectAtions... Logette"
SEMI-PRIVATE ✦

33.

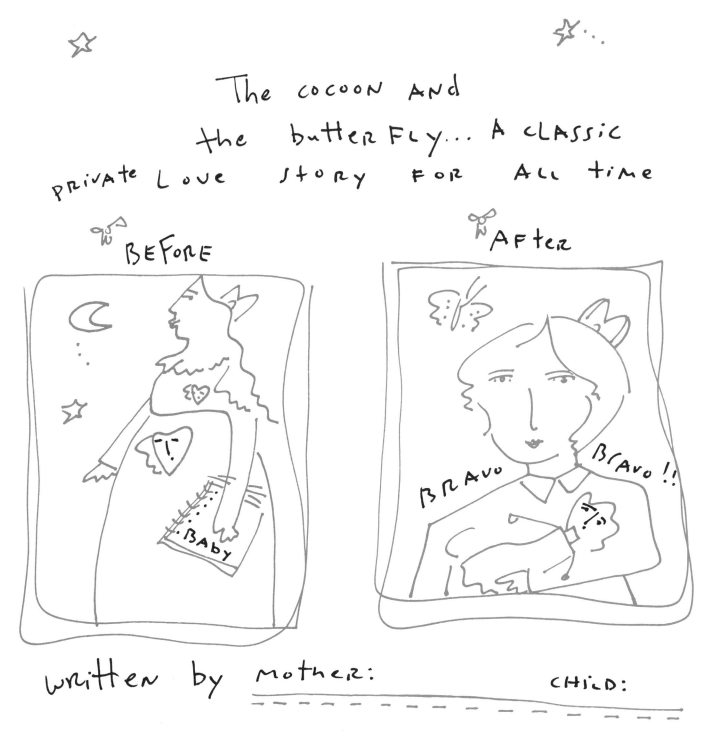

The cocoon and the butterfly... A classic private love story for all time

BEFORE

AFTER

BABY

BRAVO   BRAVO!!

written by   mother: _____   child: _____

34.

First-Aid kit... File!!!

date menu...

mom!

date
H₂O.
☑'s

Find a handsome * sturdy * envelope-like File to store some of your important data that this kit offers you, as a handy means to track your Bambino Daze. Of course you must decorate it well, with old mementos of your own baby days and grown-up days... DRAW... Color... Doodle!!

Become pals with your Doctors, Nurses And support STAFF. Bring them sweet gifts from your cookie jar or the corner bakery. Beee more than a patient on file... ZQT XOXO Ms. 1470734700 Make a list of All your questions And simple wonderments between visits. Feel entitled to CALL AFter office hours iF Need be. Your peace of MiND will Make FOR A peaceful BAmbiNO.

ARE you WRAPPED iN ANGst
oveR the physicaL biRthing?
NEVER FEAR, Aunt PeaRL is NeaR.

DARLiN, ALL you hAve to do is
look At ALL the women on eaRth
todAy... the schoolchildRen At plAy...
ANd kNow thAt youR pRize foR A
veRy tempoRARy maRAthon is
PRiceLess !!!

you'll be
just FiNe...
don't you worRy!   I PRomise !!

37.

Who, indeed, is this wise Aunt PEARL?

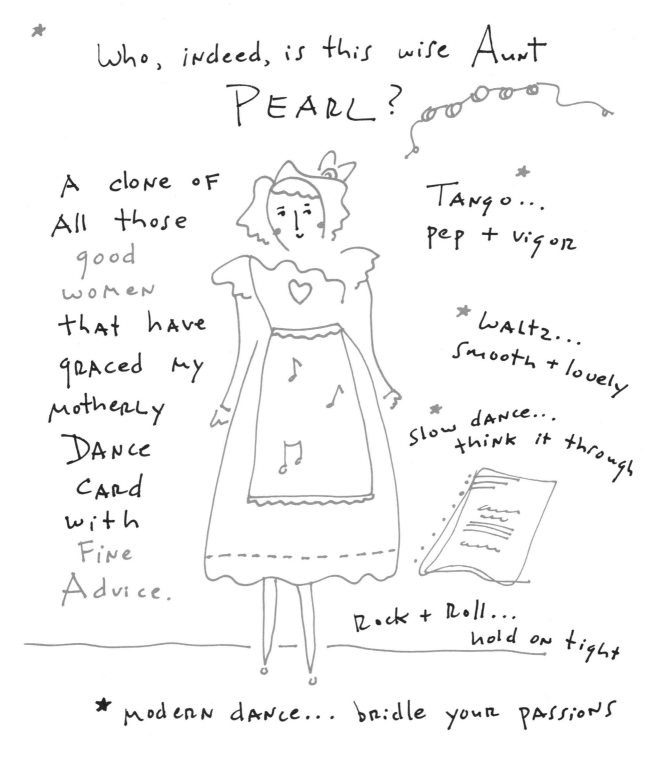

A clone of All those good women that have graced my motherly DANCE CARD with Fine Advice.

TANGO...
pep + vigor

* WALTZ...
Smooth + lovely

Slow dance...
think it through

Rock + Roll...
hold on tight

* modern dance... bridle your passions

38.

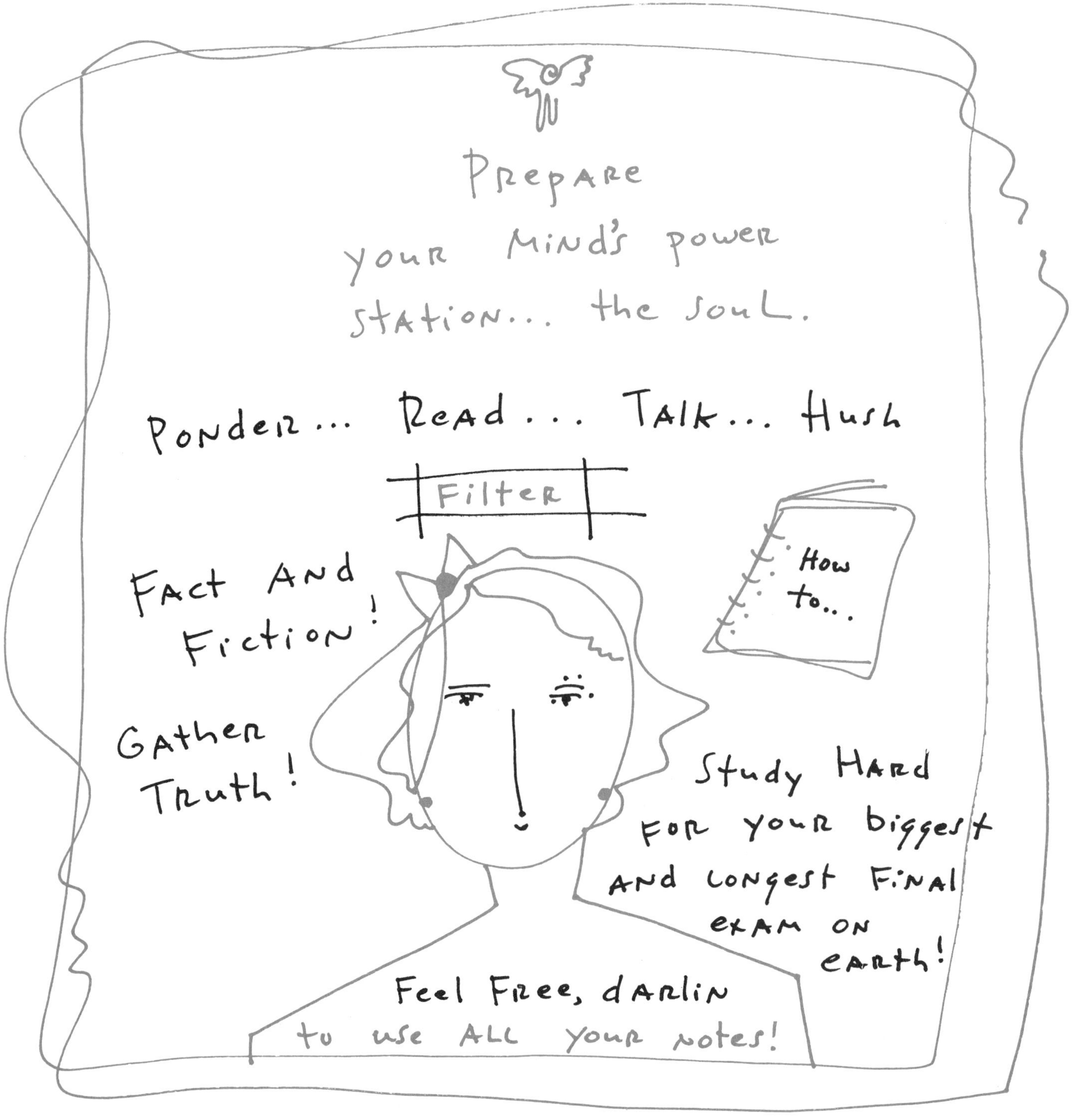
Prepare
your Mind's power
station... the soul.
Ponder... Read... Talk... Hush
Filter
Fact And Fiction!
Gather Truth!
How to...
Study Hard
For your biggest
And Longest Final
exam on
earth!
Feel Free, darlin
to use ALL your notes!

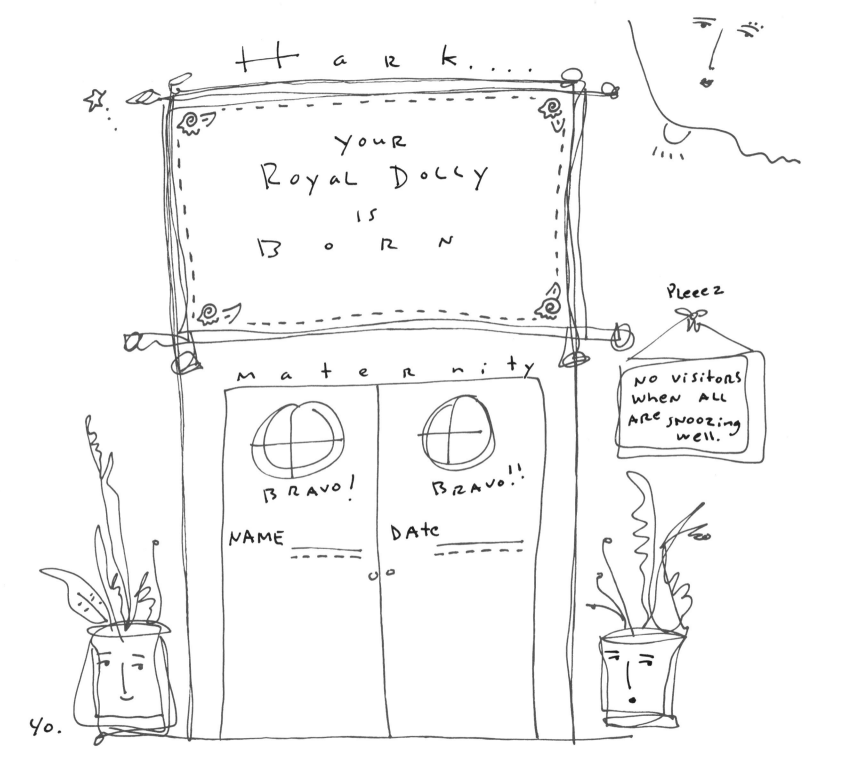

A Mother's Creed ☆
And prayer...

Please God or _____, give me
the grit And heart's bounty to care,
love, And protect this wondrous life
Let me proffer A dependence that
will later dissolve into An independence,
free of regrets And selfish guilt. Forgive
my youthful follies and guide my
stewardship of each little one's light...
into his or her own galaxy of promise.

☆ Amen!! _____

Signed   41.

<u>SOOOO</u> VERY TRUE...

"YOU HAVE NEVER FELT LOVE LIKE this iN your entire LiFe... NO MA'AM.

☆ CONGRATULATIONS, Sweet mother. Lock these moments deep inside your heart's secret museum of ALL that must REMAIN past tomorrow

☆ A WORDLESS CODE:

MAMA, I LOVE you sooo much

soooo much

How much?? THIS much...!!!

42.

DiHHo!!

mother and daughter...

WELL... Now you and your own mother both have something Really, Really in common...

Motherhood, OF course!!! Re-edit with fresh info. let your plateaus of love melt into one lush continent, with tall stands of wisdom trees and blue lakes that know no fibs.

Ask your mother questions... Darlin.

43.

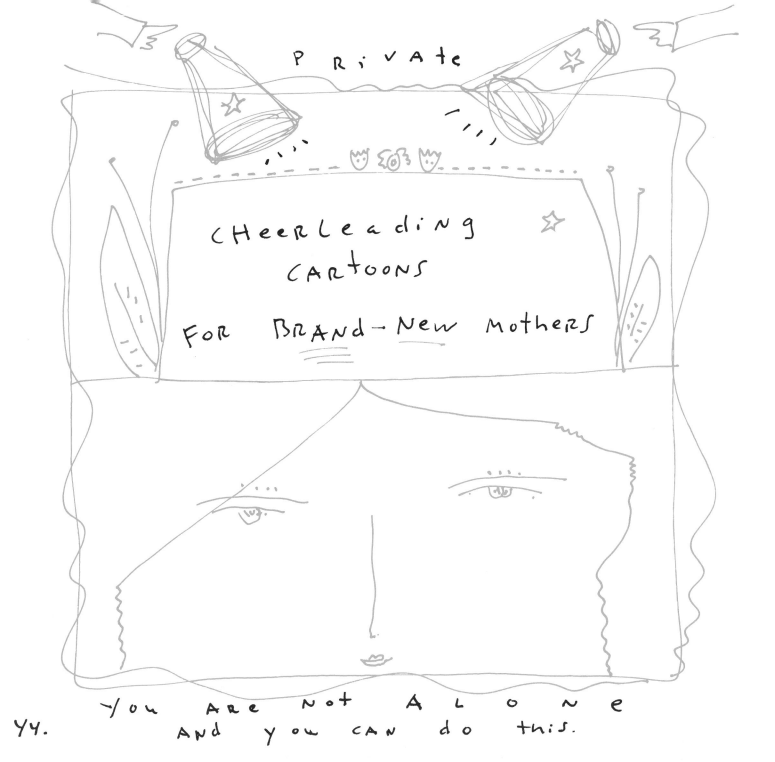

A NEW BABY does more than turn heads At the grocery or keep you up in the night, it teaches all of us to SEE the world again, For Another FIRST time.

A goood mother keeps her spectacles crystal clear And celebrates this gift.

LIFE is sooooo very grand

45.

mother dear...
COMMON sense will keep you sane
and Free...

Filter, sort, think... keep an eye
on the simple truth...

☆ Scribble together with crayons

☆ Develop a routine of basic rituals
AND stick to it!!

☆ Give your little one clear, Direct
choices: a hot dog or P.B.+ J. ???

☆ Play with them... sing... Read stories

☆ Cuddle... Stroll... Hug... Rock-a-bye!!

☆ Give them quiet, solitude, a
chance to explore alone, yet safely.

☆ Play beautiful piano music.

How to.... manage

: my very
: own
: brood...
: Love,
: mom

Experiment
w i s e l y...

Find patterns and solutions that
work for your domestic paradise.
Review the past attempts within
your own family!!! read.. listen...
swap tales with pals and strangers.
Script fresh symphonies and always
be prepared to re-edit. The only
life on earth that appears flawless
is in Orlando. (Disney, darlin...)

And even in the Magic kingdom, mama
said there'd BE DAYS like this...or did she?

From the moment of birth we each
join the humanitarian army of

FREEEdom Seekers...

While you steward your miracle
on loan, you may have to join
this particular Army's reserve unit.

4p. It is huge and full of good mothers.

Aunt Pearl Applauds the many seemingly small tasks you master so well...

BRAVO, darlin !!!

These ARE All REAlly Big Things!!
☆ spoon-feeding solid foods
☆ Mastering a healthy pattern of sleep...
☆ Protecting the crawling toddler every MOMENT!
☆ Directing the daily discoveries of motor-sensory skills !!
☆ Attending to the creative parts of life, directly tied to "Play"
☆ Nurturing the tactile senses, loving well and unconditionally xox
☆ toilet training, shoe tying, table etiquette
☆ Toy And PAl MANAgement!
☆ Delayed gratification... AN INTroduction

...Sometimes simple, repetitive chores can be a soothing balm. At the end of each day, list all that you have accomplished, and be very, very proud, indeed!!!

☆ _____

☆ _____

☆ _____

☆ _____

☆ _____

☆ _____

☆ _____

☆ the single most important... I've loved well.

Those very first years will demand that a mother become an expert interpreter of her wee one's needs and wants. Since she has no formal training in this language, she must heed her own interior "receivers" and when in doubt call THE

p e d i a t r i c i a n !!!

Good

? ? ? ? ? ? ? ?

BRAVO, sweet MAMA!

TURN OVER EVERY WORRY STONE to gather ANSWERS!

51.

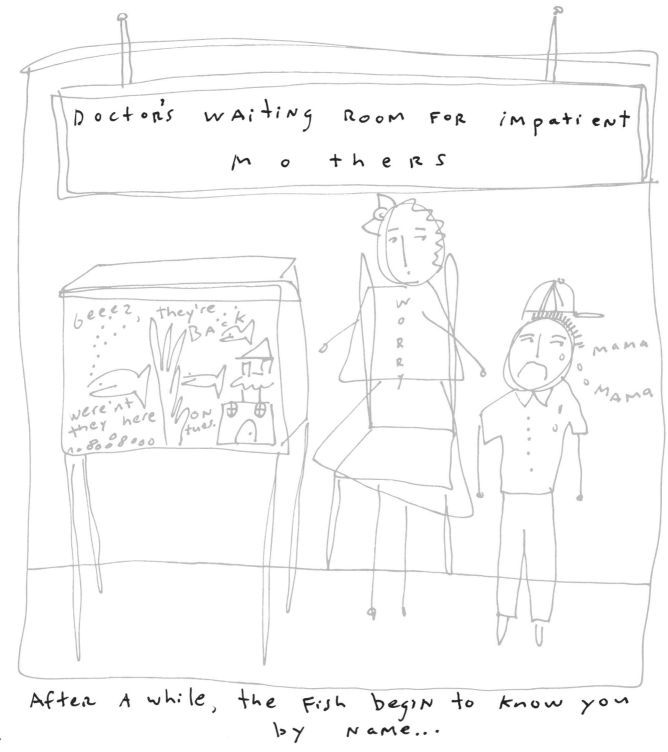

52.

FiND A DoctoR who has all of his dots connected to his HEART AND if possible see one FACE per visit. However, "groups" that prevail todAy Also Reflect a common sensibility AND they, too, can give you fine cAre. Just press great energy into this decision AND let your instincts Rule. If EVER the good Doctor leaves you feeling that All Rocks

53.

have not been turned, do what you must to prevail in the caring of your BAMBINO. Be a valiant EXPLORER. We all lean on the expertise of those who are schooled... And sometimes we must LEAN a little harder to find the remedies that Fit!!

Have we looked at all possibilities ... do we want more INFO.???

...Nudge if need be

54.

Factola:

Many good mothers are un-canonized saints... Look for them at the grocery, school parking lot, Dentist's office... If you look really hard enough and try and imagine their day's mission, much like yours, you just might see a teeny-tiny thin ┼ ┼ ┼ A L O.

How is yours glowing, dolly???...

55.

CHapter II.
The
Beginning of your Royal
☆ Stewardship

No cHiNA doll or "Tiny tears" iN plump soft rubber caN match your child's perfection ANd uniqueness. Their sweet scent of NewNess And beauty of color sAy, with every cry And wiggle: this life is strong And full. Ready or Not, dArliN, there is AN invisible umbilicAl cord thAt nothing on earth can sever (even on days when you might consider it).

During my first few weeks home from the hospital, I learned the meaning of the word "interruption". Visitors *you-who!* dropped by uNANNOUNCED, And the telephone RANG duRiNg NAp time (Let the MAchiNe FeND off those who MeAN well). You cAN try placing A note on your door that SAys politely ... xoxo

57.

CLIP AND/OR COPY!! LAMINATE FOR YOUR DOOR!!

OUR...

SWEET BABY is A-NAPPINS!!

XOX

Please come by again!!.!

Have A PURR-Fecto DAY!

58.

knock-knock

you-who!

Ring-A-ling

← These simple happenings of daily life, coupled with a little angel who tick-tocks to a separate clock, give the word "INTERRUPTION" an extraterrestrial glow.

The side effect is, of course, not a laughing matter... Fatigue is a big-league handicap to emotional and mental health. It may sound trivial... but when "MAMA" is tired, the show under the big top 59.

tends to poke along without the cotton candy and dancing bear. SNAP! SNAP!!! Yes *darling, there may be crabby moments you hope will never be videotaped or remembered. The best course is to __sleep__ whenever, wherever, for however long... and take a nice hot bath (remember your satchel of luxuries) and redefine the term

C O N T R O L. (verb)

WEBSTER'S: have the authority to regulate, direct, or dominate.

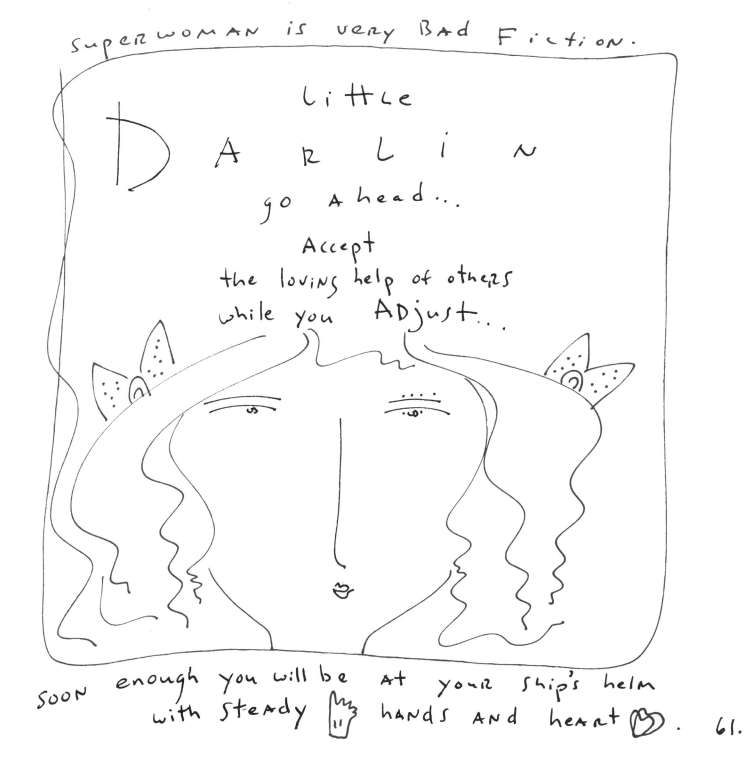

Superwoman is very bad fiction.

Little
DARLIN

go ahead...

Accept
the loving help of others
while you ADjust...

soon enough you will be at your ship's helm
with steady hands and heart. 61.

Bend like a willow. Take each day as a mini-mountain B. H. expedition of "Baby and Home" management. When you feel like a good cry, let the rivers flow. Create a country of sister lakes if you must. Do not expect to graduate from "Girl Scout" to "Mother Scout" overnight. (Eat some of their cookies) though. Like all new frontiers, "getting a

62.

HANDLE" on A "pocket full of Jingling Dimes" takes AN exceptional Heroine. And you are certainly A fine candidate!!!

Let's pretend your heart's mind AND soul ARE WRApped iN AN invincible cloak of CoRTen steel... one that Allows the iNsiqnificant bothers of your bizee dAys AND Nights to Roll off iNto "NoT important" land. Hold that beautiful

63.

baby tight, look deeply into those trusting eyes, 👁|👁 Breathe A sigh of calm And sing A semi-original Lullaby!!!...

♫ With my Maggie, AN early delivery iN "emergency" fashion, I borrowed the tune from "Pretty Baby" And fussed with custom lyrics for this 5-pound, 10-ounce Angel.

MAKE up youR own tune!

IF you ARE A Homemade DivA (the best kind), explore simple tunes that are adapted to your audience. No doubt there will be RAVE reviews from within your CRADled ARMS. Remember that this first wave of time outside of your castle needs a bit of "bridging", As two hearts, minds, and bodies work to settle in Lovingly!!! (And our divine LANDLORD says, "Howdy, Folks... WELCOME TO EARth.) Touch... hold... sing... laugh... Hum... ROck-A-byE ALL Blues AWAY... with soft messages of love and comfort and a safety net that ENDURES most ★ tightrope faux pas. Sometimes a spiritual journey comes without a passport, motherhood is one of those.

Aunt Pearl, a golden friend and mentor of mine, would stop by every now and then. She never had children of her own and, after marrying twice, moved onto a more singular island in time. She was lovely to look at... neatly kept with a silk snood at the nape of her neck and ivory

stockings sporting seams as right as rain. They
came from one of her "New York city"
catalogs. Always, she would call first and
while she sat with us in the living room's
best chair, her mother's locket-watch, pinned
to her suit jacket, was flipped up often toward
her studious eyes. Pearl never overstayed,
undertipped, or paid debts a moment
too late.
             On that first visit she brought
a small gift, wrapped   in a frail

swatch of lace, tied with a tussie-
mussie of fresh lavender pansies. It
was a leather book of empty pages.
Her inscription (always in a thick Fountain
pen of sienna ink) read:

- -

Nancy dear... Every day in life
is a fresh page... You be the co-author
of this mother-child sojourn and always
remember that you do NOT pen this
new life to perfection... only aspire to
pen your role in it, as best as one
soul can.

68.

Goodness, how I loved Aunt Pearl. Everyone needs their very own personal cheerleader to nudge them on. And we all need to serve our turn doing the same... For New mothers, especially... I cheer you on with pep and gusto !!! When your stroller crosses the path of another, remember to do the same!! This can be as simple as a kind smile that says, "I know exactly how your semi-muddled day is going !!! keep up the

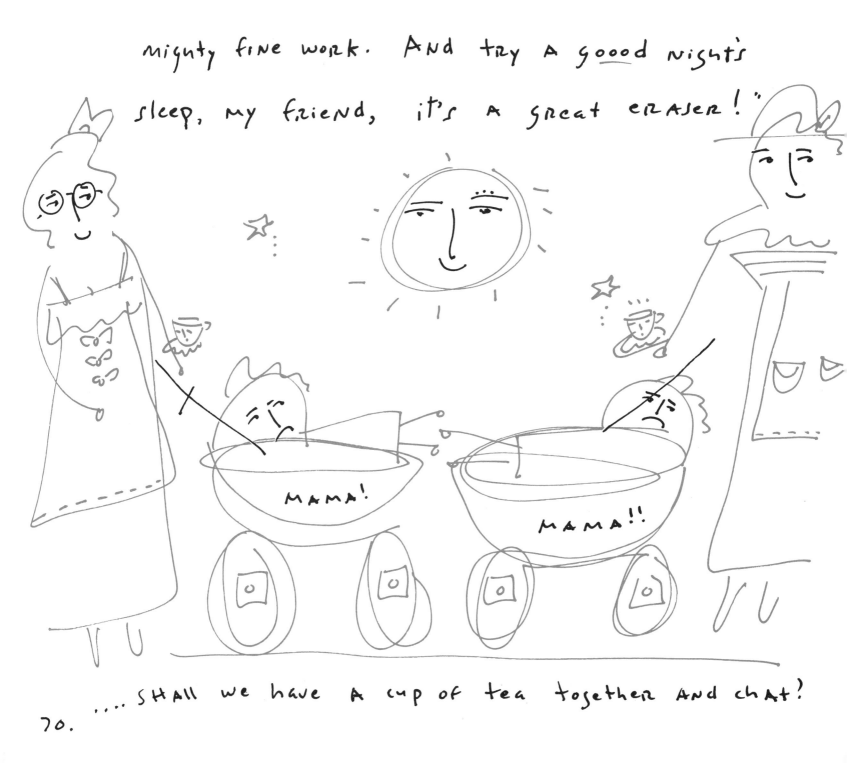

MASTER
THE
ART
OF
III.

DISCIPLINE ?

Lovingly
delivered with a
touch of resolve and
forgiveness... And, darlin,
always
married to CONSISTENCY!

71.

Discipline...

The method should be firm, kind, and non-violent. Restraining a child from self-destruction requires a relentless heart and even mind. As the ability to reason enters your domain, consider the Round Table approach or a Gandhi-type delivery. Your Home sweet home within four walls exists a small prototype of a nation, really... May peace rule your

L i v e s

together.

EARLY .... EARLY.... BAMBINO days...

Your very best resource when "they" Are young And without "REASON" is to cobble A formidable Fort of "Routine" with moats to protect them from the ill winds of fate And their endearing NON-REASONABLE selves.

☆ Guard them in both visible And invisible ways.

73.

ALL FAULTS IN LIFE WILL HAVE CONSEQUENCES, SOME FAIR AND OTHERS NOT WHEN YOU ARE JUDGE AND JURY OF YOUR YOUNG BROOD, * Select RATIONAL ONES. THAT teach AND do NOT destroy the human spirit... Measure your POWER WITH A CARE THAT TAKES THE CHILD'S LIFE MORE seriously THAN MOMENTARY circumstances.

gosh, that's TUFF!!

mmm... but possible!!

74.

✦ From the moment of your baby's very first breath a battle begins. This battle is titled "You are not the boss of me... I am the boss of me." Of course, my dear

✳ mother, some day when all is right and well, your child will ✦ win. Until then it is, indeed,

75.

up to you to wage a war that
only a mother's heart can
design. A fight for balance,
safety, and a final freedom
that will set your angel off
in flight to a wondrous life.
A life you partnered.

My friend Mary Jo, a
schoolteacher, pointed out one

LUCKY CHARM ... In her calm voice via telephone, she said, "NANCY, All children really want and need is a loving measure of CONsistency... order ...clearly drawn fences, if you may". Like a good TEACHER, a mother must draft a PLAN to get the job

77.

done And stick to it like bubble gum on Cinderella's glass slipper. She deftly drafts sturdy lesson plans to carry her little ones well into the LAnd of Grown-Ups. This is very tricky because we Are All creatures of comfort and habit... with

a strong will for whim and

pronto gratification. A mother

must marry many conflicting

passions in order to ensure a

healthy life and future for

her borrowed prize.

The remarkable twist

79.

to these lesson plans is
that many of us "mothering"
are still in the process of
growing up ourselves, weaving
personal safety nets and dream-quilts!
Could it be that this little
one is here as a T.A.
(teaching assistant) for a course

Not yet offered at Harvard??

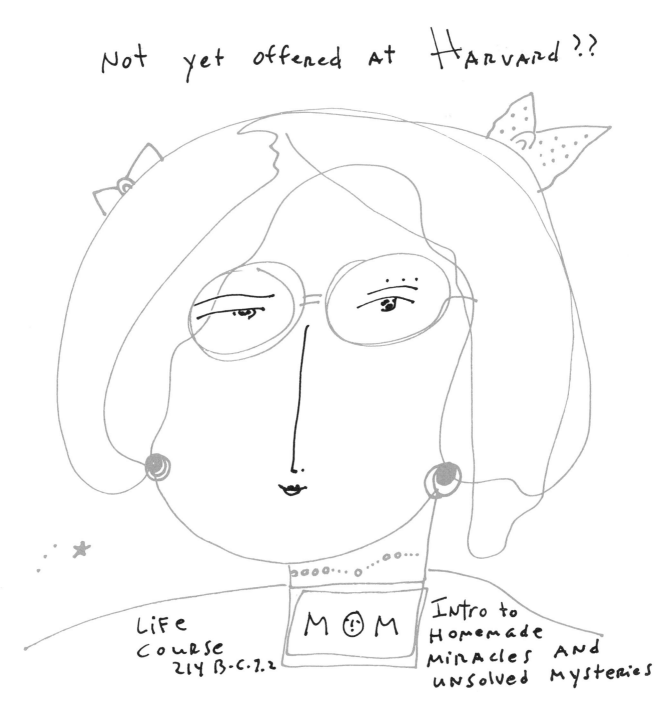

LiFe
course
214 B.C.7.2

MOM

Intro to
Homemade
Miracles and
unsolved Mysteries

81.

sometimes...

it's best to maximize the little things because they are often cloaked in costumes of insignificance to hide their HUGENESS.

Do not be Fooled!!!

☆ Teach your child simple things well and applaud their daily mastering, step by step.

☆ Imagine miniature trophies inscribed "I think I can... I know I can," kept close to their hearts' memory in time.

Honesty

is a young child's gift to all those near.

They RALLY and illuminate the truth... like meteors do the ink black night. Mother them well in a blanket of the same, and PROFFER a spiritual bounty for all of their GROWN-UP-HOOD !!

xoxo

CHAPTER IV.
School DAze...Taxi DAze... HAt DAze

MAMA

A,B...Z

Too Too Much, dolly? You CAN do this!

"Getting to know Kiddo... And your sweet Kiddo getting to know the world"

Not all mothers have kept those old-fashioned Albums of their child's first lock snipped At the kitchen sink or the single tooth that led one to believe in cash for personal loss. Most, however, Remember well that very first day of SCHOOL. The preparation And most significantly the feeling

85.

that takes charge unannounced of your HEART and tear ducts as you drive away. The streets and trees, stoplights, and curbs seem to say softly, "It's OK, Mom... it's really OK".

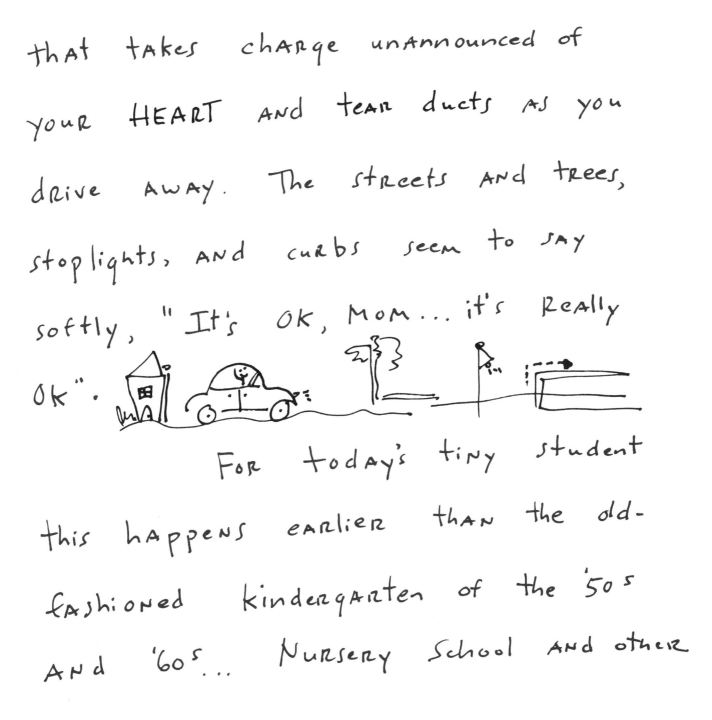

For today's tiny student this happens earlier than the old-fashioned kindergarten of the '50s and '60s... Nursery School and other

Pre-schools are often a blend ⭐...
of sophisticated play and discovery.
This, too, is another example of
how hurried our culture can be
to graduate our young, Pronto,
into the perpetual school of Adulthood. ⭐ But for those moms who
have 2½ or so hours of freedom,
this time is at first teary and

soon oh-so-liberating. Most likely these semi-free moments are spent frugally, like pennies... running errands and attending the business of homemaking, without your little one's company. Walking and moving about with an empty hand and hip to match can be a dreamy gift, darlin!! space When the time is up, your TAxi joins the

motor PARAde of moms Awaiting

A full Report, pRAying that

their bambino's Review is more

happy than just so-so. Luckily

for me, I Recall Nice cheshire

smiles And construction-made turkey

hats that often were worn until

bed time. Days like those first

days of dropping off one's heart, to be picked up later, will fill your motherhood pockets many a time... with the miracle of LEtting Go. A comforting remembrance

for me of those school daze was

...* FINALLY Feeling

like I was not too bad at my

mothering career and that I was indeed the boss (sort of). That is not to say it was serenely silky and wrinkle-free. No, it was a daily power struggle to polish the veneer of ordered chaos, while learning the true meaning of two words I had never paid much attention to: interruption and unfinished.

:* The "wearing Too many Hats"
syndrome for mothers has always
been around. It's just
that with our generation's recent
experiment of "Bringing Home some
of the Bacon and Brie, while
running a Mother Goose compound,
*
sporting a Victoria's Non-secret
ensemble", more Hats than could

92.

could fit into YANkee StAdium
have been woRN. This RUNAWAY
tRAiN CRuNCH has caught
the best of us dREAming At
dusk of A moRe merciful clock.
Well, dAnlin, the "TIMEX" foe
would glAdly bow to your
wishes if it were At All
possible...

so...so soRRY!! There's

only one solution to your pickle

And that is to clean your

chapeau closet... ASAP! Study

all those snappy caps ,

dressy bonnets , tattered

berets ... and resign a

few, wrapped in respectful papers,

to a quiet bandbox xox.

wear your dreams, one at a time

with the highest honor, and

crown them jewels of precious

REALity!

When I look back into

my fuzzy crystal ball ? of

longish days that vanished

David Copperfield style, I do remember certain hats that were oh _so_ important!! These I would lovingly stitch and embroider all over again... See what you think, dolly.

In our sparkling little town, a sweet shop, THE PARIS CANDY, with Tiffany lanterns and mahogany booths, sat smartly in the middle of Main Street near a lonesome stoplight. Mrs. Harriet Patterson, a MAGNIFICENT mother of sons and daughters and then some, purveyed real works of art in chocolate and caramel and peppermint.

→Ribbon candy

After school, and well before, we and other townsfolk escaped flat gray days and celebrated sunny ones at THE PARIS CANDY STORE. Sometimes the Hoover had to just wait a bit for its daily exercise! My three could rest assured that a grilled cheese, hot cocoa, or cherry phosphate,

Along with paper and crayons, would turn any little slumps into satin rainbows! Mrs.

Patterson often sat with us and I, very happy to chat with some-one over seven or eight, loved the company. We covered more worlds than our downtown Main Street ever afforded. Sometimes a diamond sits right outside your window looking for a spot to shine atop

a trusty sill. On some

occasions my girls would stroll their

best dolls to The PARIS CANDY Store

and sit them in a high chair for

a pretend butterscotch sundae.

As Mitt, the big brother, grew

older and became a Little Leaguer,

those dolls were left at home, until

days when Mitt was away at
practice.

strike 2

One of the gifts from
Mrs. Patterson to us was the
mantra she lived by: "If
you must do something anyway,
no matter how unpleasant, go on
and do it with a smile, darlin."

Her life was sometimes a non-
saccharine tapestry of heartful

toil and bodily wear. When she walked purposefully upon the mosaic floor toward the back kitchen of copper cauldrons and blue flames, her silvering hair framed a smile that held deep chasms full of secrets only a mother can keep.

This hat... the " TEA-PARTY imaginary Hat"... I devote to Harriet. She, like you and me, might have wished to alter some facts to fiction. However, with a gentility that comes from sharing a spot of sweet tea, dollies dressed for the Ritz, and the exchanging of a hopeful wisdom, life can deliver ribboned presents that smile back, along any Main St.

103.

TEA-PARTY IMAGINARY Hat

HAVE MOMENTS of pretend, in between RUNNING AND fetching AND waiting...Brew A pot of teA AND cozy up to your REAL LiVE doll BABies... while you mAY!

P.C.

Another favorite hat was (and
still is) "Home Art Teacher." This is a job

that requires only one, yes, only one
propensity... A LOVE OF PLAY. I have
No doubt that you are well-endowed

in memory and practical spirit, just create a humble or so Ho-loft-like spot in your nest for coloring, drawing, cutting, and pasting. Even a portable shoe box tucked in a cupboard, ready to transform your kitchen table into a magic carpet, will do! As you develop your skills (see THE ARTFUL SPIRIT...CRAFTY HOBBIES TO GIFT WRAP your LiFe) there are many HANdy tools to add to your HOME CURRICULUM. The first class should be "Scribbling 101". With large

paper And classic crayons, let your

wee one loop And dip And jot their

interior Map for All the world to see.

Find A way to weave this work

into An evolving exhibit throughout the

house. Consider the fridge, doors, corkboards,

And Plexiglas frames As prime gallery space

to brilliantly display their "Picasso-esque"

Rumblings!! As they scribble their way

toward more configurations, consider personalized Christmas cards and other reproducible items (e.g. notepads). These are definitely "Hallmarks" worth saving and an enormous boost to the child's sense of what within must be spent, loved, and kept!!

"A" is for Always

i Luv You mom!e

i Really do

Oh yes... And A "must" chapeau during those school Daze: "THE Mother Nature" CAP. Let your babies see the

A d j e n t u r e ....

R O A M

outside world iN A very Annie Oakley — Daniel Boone way... * EARly!! This can happen without FARAWAY travel or American Express dough-re-me. Soak your baby-child's "sponge" of wonder

with ☼ the wind AND snow AND

RAin And sun. ☀ Find A

PARk 🪑 ... beach ⛵ ...

Meadow 🌾 Leave youR

choRes behind (weARing A MRs.

PAtteRson smile) and scoot AwAy

fRom home to discoveR God's best

And most sacRed cAthedRAl...

110.

the out-of-doors, where your little one will need no pacifier or couture gear to bathe in clouds of peace. Let the blue jays and sparrows yackety-yack while you and your pal marvel. This offer is FREE... knows no expiration date... and most certainly may never be found at WALMART.

lll.

And you know, sweetheart, in your life you will spend more than enough time at the checkout counter. Sooo please check out your "mother nature" cap... often!! And when you do, linger, darlin... linger.

Then there is your PoliceWoman Hat!! This one rarely takes a nap.

Fair Play

It is your sense of right and wrong, and its enforcement, that tells many a true story daily, and in a profound way scripts all of our lives!

*

Dispense your messages with

A gentleness that tells them

that no matter the error,

it is their behavior or choice

that may be faulty... not their

total being. Consequences are life's

badges of participation. While at

your command post of the mighty

114.

earthly mother (being judge and jury) take great care to see 👓 that the punishment does not swallow the spirit whole and till fertile ground for more weeds.

My good friend and mentor, Mr. Maury Hahn, a brilliant CPA and sage sifter of "Family Fact and Fiction" told me once that every conversation * is a negotiation

115.

AND that it is critical to sort
the little potatoes from the big
potatoes (I think this goes back
to the Depression Era). Well... remember
that WRONG AND Right need very little
negotiation but that GRAY AREAS
may. And the "potato" rule is an
excellent way to sort through
what is indeed of most importance...
You cannot address EACH potato
with the SAME Lens or Focus. When

116.

you don your "Policewoman" Hat...
(see page 113) back its wizardry up
with a good night's sleep, vitamins,
and a teapot tempered with a
healthy spout. If your "anger
gauge" approaches the "WARNING
ZONE", take an immediate respite:
walk outdoors... clear your lungs
under a tall pine tree... ride a
bike to NEW ZEALAND... or make

117.

outRAgeous FACES in a
mirror... For only you to see.
In other words, take your
tempest to Moses on a
mountaintop high... Let it spiral
up to your best Friend in
a Quest for Help !!.!

OH, dear God... I'm
A little lost here...

S. O. S.

Hush
darlin...
I'll
help you,
you'll see.

118.

Ready for another headdress, dolly?

This one is the "Fairy Tale to Fact" chapeau.

MAke-believe | Reality

when your children are tiny, their world will be framed by rich walls of pretend and myth. This, a glorious spell, will fade over time as

119.

Reality moves Right in. As you

begin with lap-time Readings

of Cinderella and wind in the

willows, Fast Forward in your

motherly mind to a "plan" for

bridging

lovely waters of fantasy to

those that may require life jackets.

One mother I knew, from

120.

college days, Applied her scientifically
Astute mind to this task by
simply loading All Facts of REALity
into one long sermon when her
young Einstein entered the DOOR
of Reason. This was some
sermon!! I suggest A spoon-feeding
(without visible utensils) of Reality,
so As not to send their Fairy
Tale Hopes And Dreams to Another

GALAXY... This can be done with deft LASER precision in loving doses, not all at once or too much at a time. Remember your early days of the high chair, when more Gerber products came out those sweetheart lips than stayed in?? Well... work with your salty truths like a master sculptor... and retain the natural beauty of their first dreams, which by the way, was the first

122. Real spiritual nutrition you bestowed.

A keeper

Do not EVER give this chapeau to Goodwill. It is a classic that EVERY-
ONE loves... EVEN you, mother dear...

Remember???

the MOMMIE - NURSE HAT!!!

A cup of chicken broth, vicks rubbed on
a tight chest, the HAND on the
Forehead. Visits to the doctors, phone
calls for reports... CHecking in the
still of the night through a cracked door.
Bless this Hat!

123.

Another good hat that is a great problem solver... (tested in many history books) is the

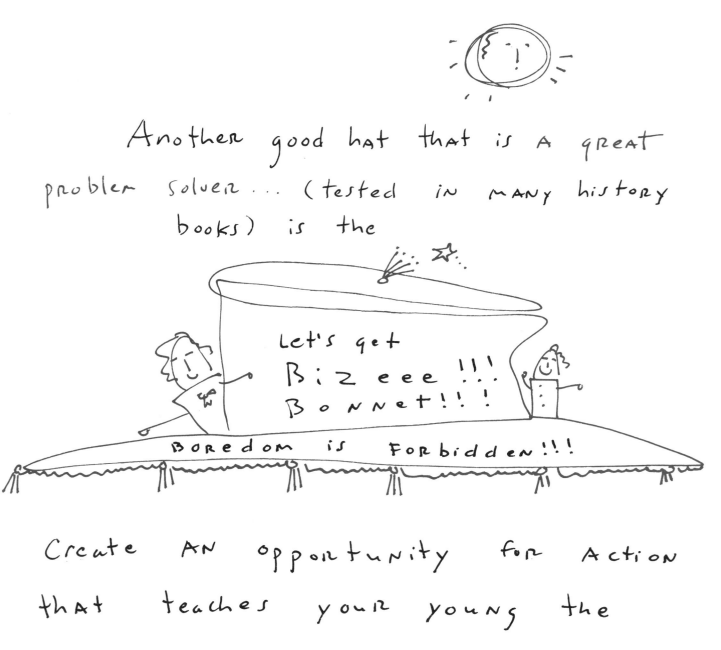

Let's get Bizeee!!! Bonnet!!!

Boredom is Forbidden!!!

Create an opportunity for action that teaches your young the pleasures of goodness. In making oatmeal cookies or dancing in the living room with a broom as your partner... picking up sticks in the yard and piling them carefully for kindling <u>or</u> for no reason at all!! when there are "blue" ♫ days this hat can be magic and like a balm; "things" will seem and feel, perhaps, not so bad. let your child know

*...

this MAGIC

As a part of everyday life that is not video - scripted. Take heed in how much and what passive entertainment combats the simple joys of the Bizeee Bonnet!! Give a visible boost to participation in sports, team projects at home, and helping a neighbor or not - so - stranger on the street. Doing nice things can chase worry

126.

And woe out your backyard and down the yellow brick road. Let the wicked witch deal with all those "boring" details... you and your Bambinos... just Get Bizeee!

xoxo

All recipes are not the same...

Select your ingredients wisely and VoiLA!!! timely blue-ribbon winners will doll-up your days together!

MORE
H a t s

you MAY wish to wear...

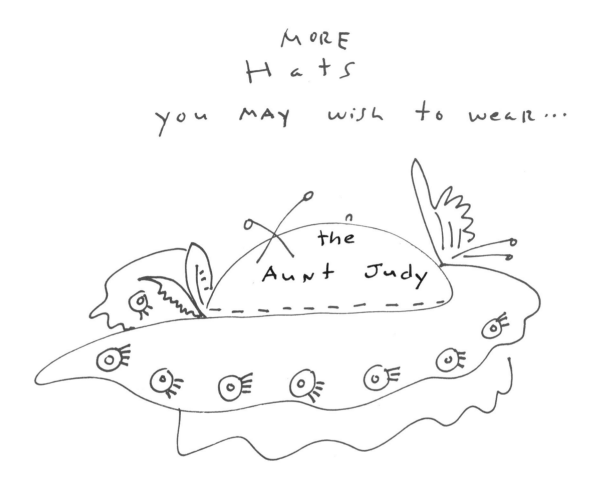

Named After My best friend At 23
Market Street since 1970. She
carries her own Angelic gifts of
unconditional love, for All Family

And enough friends to fit into a teeny-tiny country. This mother And businesswoman gift wraps each holiday and birthday present... (tons of them, too), writes wonderful old-fashioned letters, and still cooks blue-chip recipes. In addition to living with a dear respect for "rituals" And community she has spent a lion's share of her life listening to me. No small task. This chapeau comes with a sweet dotted swiss veil and hat pins.

129.

"The Sister Kathy Hat" is a solid Derby of wisdom, calm, and very

It helps that she has a big degree in counseling.

wholesome laughter. Sisters can often be the glue that holds an entire family together. This is a gift that shines

130.

best in adulthood, when life is
not a tea party of mud pies
and sand castles... if you know
what I mean. This Derby is
worn by an expert listener with
an eye that helps you see other-
wise missed perspectives. I love
you, Kathy.

131.

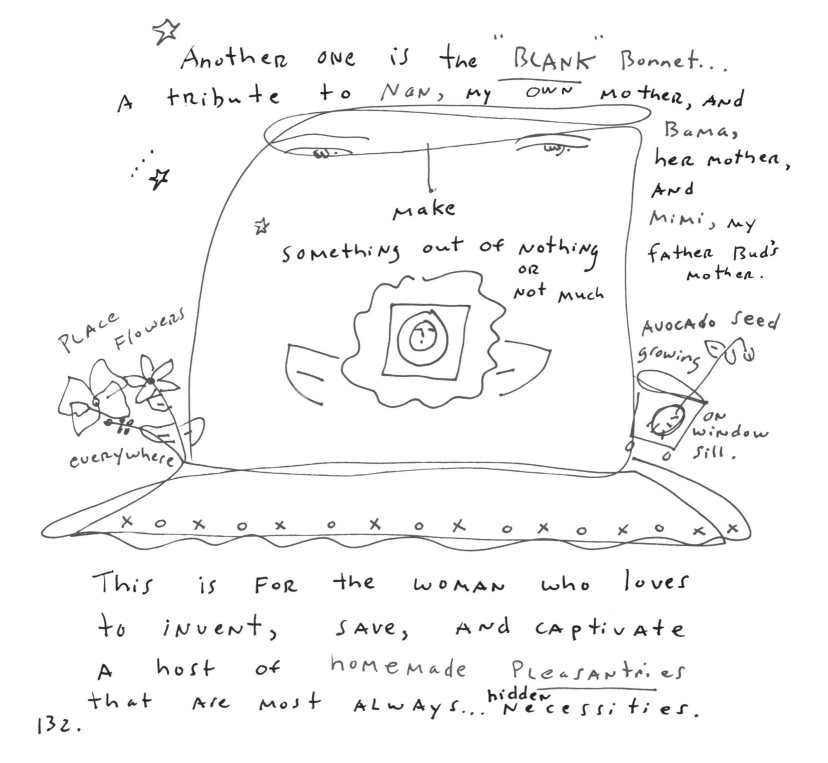

Another one is the "BLANK" Bonnet...
A tribute to Nan, my OWN mother, And
Bama, her mother, And Mimi, my father Bud's mother.

make
something out of nothing
or
not much

PLACE Flowers
everywhere

AVOCADO seed growing
on window sill.

x o x o x o o x o x o x o x o x x

This is FOR the woman who loves
to invent, save, and captivate
A host of homemade Pleasantries
that are most always... hidden Necessities.

132.

Another... Fine Hat ...

FINER THAN FROG HAIR...

the Mary Jo Heroine Bonnet

This hat is dedicated to women who, while battling nasty demons of physical persuasion (the "C" word or others just as arduous) carry on a life of mothering that rarely sends a wrinkle of this "truth"

133.

through the rest of the family whose heart

Aches with the knowing of her daily

mountaineering. ★ It is so darn

tough to be A good mother... without

other Roadblocks!! Bravo to those who

wear Mary Jo's HEROINE BONNET. You

teach the rest of us well.

XOXO

Well enough about HAts... Except
to mention those that I have ⭐...
so happily given away to
"Goodwill Heaven" :

I.   The cocktail party Hat...

II. The Town Crier Hat...
     (too much gossip is bad for many)

III. The "I can do more than

     Anyone " Volunteer Hat...

IV. The "I can Fix everyone's
     trouble" Hat ... (Family therapist)

⭐

135.

V. The "Flirting is Fun" Hat
(Ask ex-wives about this one)

VI. The "CHURCH DEPENDENCY" Hat
(leave All to holy waters)

So, darling... the best First-
Aid at this "School Daze... Taxi Daze"

pocket of mothering is to fret less

over unfinished details... select your

wardrobe of chapeaus keenly... And

Love your brood like a Fem-Grizzly does her
Cubs.

On those days when you feel as

though you are trapped inside a wooden keg

About to embark over Niagara Falls,

I say... I know the feeling. It's

one no words can touch... And

somehow your little roly-poly keg

will reach a calm pool, After each

And every Wild ride!!! It's a

Miracle Really... A mother lode

Miracle.

wow...
Not again...

137.

When your eyes become puddles of

unfinished tasks,   and your mind

is weary of traveling a road

that shows no sure sign of arrival,

read this token of a mother's

truth:

every ···☆··· day
your precious job is to give life
itself... there is no <u>finish line</u>,
darling... there is only this
"miracle" to star in, witness,
and love back...

c o m p l e t e l y.

138.

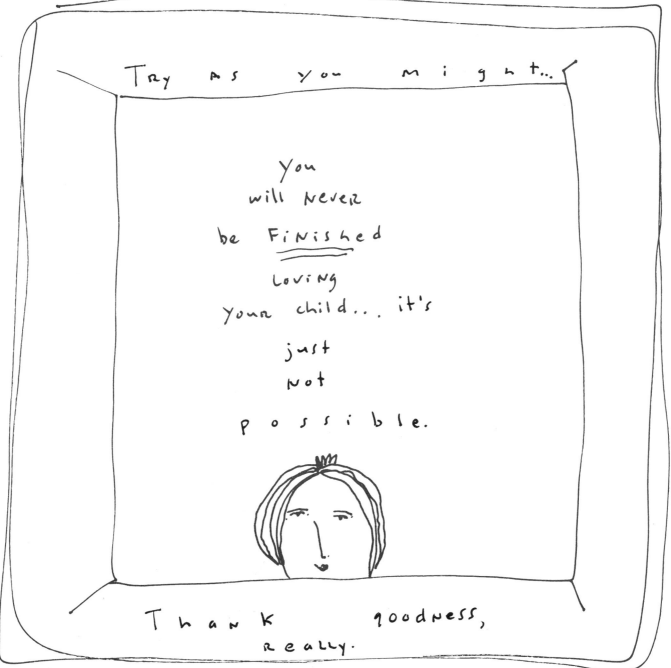

Try as you might...

You
will never
be FiNished
loving
your child... it's
just
Not
possible.

Thank goodness, really.

139.

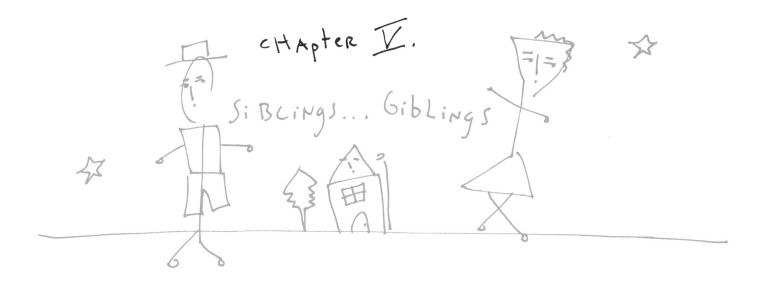

CHAPTER V.

Siblings... Giblings

"Mom... who do you love the most???" is a sure sign that your nest occupants are reassessing their original territory. Raising a family involves more than having a dog and call-waiting. It refers to a group... batch... bunch... gang. This Multiplicity leads to more of everything: milk... toilet paper... squabbles... victories... laughs... And A Huge contest over who is your Favorite. A mother of eleven told me recently that her mother of nine would answer that question this way: "My favorite is the one who has left home and comes to visit or the one who has been ill and gets better." Isn't that just the

141.

best?? I tell my three that of course I love them all the same And that they are indeed each my Favorites. That is A must. They may Not feel it or believe it, but from A mother's Registry of Honor it is A must.

When you mindfully imagined your "Family - To - Be", A christmassy picture might have Appeared in living color, with A sweetness of sharing

And love that glows like 🍬 candy canes

lit by bright red, blue, and orange

bulbs atop pine needles. This is

the dream that led you to the

altar of mothering once again. Now

that some of you are well into

number two or three or more,

that cozy picture around the tree

has probably gone to Tibet. *ooops*

   I'll WAGER ... you've already

discovered that each little one
is not a carbon copy of the
one before, and that the
routine that was customized
for Susie or Billy isn't exactly
working as well for Todd. This
is your golden time to shine like
the moon over Indiana pumpkin
patches!! Yes, you must re-edit...
without abandoning all that is

essential... Remaining impartial and fair and steady. Oh, you are so very wonderful and good at free-falling!!! Dancing this sibling JIG (BANANA peel) in bare feet with your wits, dreaming of Club Med for couples, is tricky.

Watch, like a detective, those other "Family Batches" around you and ask your own mother questions. Try to remember your early feelings as a sibling-gibling!!! This info 145.

will fill your mental notebook so that the maternal student you Are can put All good tips to practice And dismiss the rest. There is, of course, the emotional notebook that your heart monitors daily. Try to have quiet moments of consultation between HEART And MIND. Inevitably they Are co-captains of your domestic ship... And Neither Must be slighted.

This summer while At Ruby Creek, I witnessed A lesson of practical faith that is a real keepsake. Earlier in the spring a robin had built a nest in a log's niche above a screen door. One afternoon, the nest was finally full of three "chirpers" clad in scruffy fuzz-buntings, sporting JUMBO beaks that popped up and down with out respite. No mother robin to be seen, I thought about my next possible job as a fly catcher... but ALAS there she came, full-breasted and proudly trailing a juicy worm (HUGE)

147.

from her beak. I stood on a chair
from a safe distance and wondered
how she would evenly distribute this
NOONDAY lunch to her hungry CREW.
Surely, she would find a way to chop
that worm up three ways. No, sir.
The one robin in the center was
really going to town with a "birdie tizzie fit"
and, lo and behold, the mother (after pause)
gracefully let that whole long worm
become a solitary gift. She must have

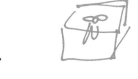

148.

felt, for good mothering reasons, that in that moment... one baby needed more. She certainly flew additional missions and fulfilled the needs of her other two. But don't you see??? Sometimes there will be patches, short INtense ONES, that might demand more from you and others. AND YES, one child at any given time or for a whole lifetime may need to be fed some things first. That is not to mean, ever, that they are your favorite... It means ONLY that their PARTICULAR prescription of need places them slightly in the front of some lines. How I pray that someday all those little ones standing behind watching and waiting will know that it was really just that. A life-survival mode to keep the family whole... because losing A CHILD is A mother's most dire fear. Hush now... And decide as best you can which of your robins, in this blink of time, needs you the most... And go.

150.

Your very own Pulitzer Prize Afternoon...

Play again with a Butterfly's love of flight. Revisit your keen ☆ imagination ☆ and pack a picnic for the beach along the shore. Tell stories aloud, building them word by word... WAVE by WAVE... ones that say, "I love you FOR-EVER AND A SEASHELL"

151.

P.S.

When the in-fighting becomes a warring
nightmare,

★ separate your little ones
so that a calm pause
may lead to temporary
PEACe!!

Little
Miss
Muffet

A simple nap... time-out play...
or hushed nursery rhyme can
do wonders.

152.

TEENAGE
unsolved mysteries

...Fasten your Heart's seat belt...
sweet good mother that
you ARE !!

☆

Remember this well: Any captain can
steer a ship over calm seas. It's
only the wise, valiant one who
leads her ship Atop wild waters to
safe sugar Beaches...

153.

Chapter VI.

THE Alien Plateau....

t e e n a g e r s

If you are one who claims you were a great teen, no trouble to the family, and now have your own teenagers who are also ducky... please call me at 1·800·776-3739 For a Free gift!! Congratulations... perhaps a Ripley's Believe-It-or-Not STudy is in order! Maybe you are Amish...

or have just moved to the U.S.A.

from a quiet European Village yet to have Television.

Nevertheless, BRAVO to you!!

It is my "listening" collection of other's voices AND EXPERIENCES that CONFIRMS: for A vast majority, this is the concentrated time of parenting, during which A mother may visualize running away from her

VERY OWN HOME to BELIZE... where She would call herself tutti-Fruiti-Irene AND weave bAsKets for happy-go-lucky tourists. Most women I have known never really do this. They may have A series of private "breakdowns," develop NERVOUS habits, cry frequently (which is then blamed on hormones... WRONG), or take mini-VACATIONS At A _Bed And Breakfast_ where they stay in their ROOM, reading self-Help books.

This plateau can, like Boot Camp, either make or break you and that goes for the rest of the family. If you have considered going back to church, this is a great time to do so.

Also...

Check into your health insurance policy to see if there is coverage for therapy. Even though mothers are gifted problem solvers, there may ★ come a time when you need outside

"Interpreters" or even a bit more. The safety net you've spun might need to be expanded and reinforced T E M P O R A R I L Y!!

May I fortify your net with a First-Aid Remedy? look back long enough to know you are doing a Fine job... refresh your collection of hats... add a few like the

VIGILANT surprise watcher.

This is one that, if you can only imagine, increases your already astute sensors to the state and needs of your child. Remember when they were tiny and not yet skilled in ENGLISH? Well... sometimes these teen years are "RETRO" in that way, and once again "reading" them is, mmm... difficult. So... listen harder...

159.

while watching them closely AND of course loving them No matter what. xoxoxo

Heighten your AgeNdA!! Review All the good And wonderful parts of your relationship And prepare to ARMOR your heart of hearts... BiG Time!!!

When you first embarked on this journey, much joy came from the "loving" BACK...

MoM!

<u>Nice</u> hugs and huge grins and soft, dear times, when snuggling told each of you a love story from above. <u>Please</u> hold on to all of this... In many ways, those early years anchored your sense of worth and ability to mother. All was pretty well, especially at night, when the house was still and they were safely tucked into bed, right down the hall! <u>Hectic</u>... but safe, your

161.

domain was. Now, the TEEN climate may alter this landscape and you must again re-edit your mothering in order to carry on. To help you recall those steadier days place sweet memory photos all about!! Leave your teenagers "love" notes... Sometimes the toneless benign post-Its are a good reminder of your devotion.

There is a player of enormous power in this varsity game

of REALity And the daily Recruiting
of your Angel to be less than whole. Try out by
TRy OUT.   It is the culture...
And like A shakespearean Play, LiFe's
tug of wAr will be between dArkness
And light, Always, darlin.

          You're not to be A helpless
Nanny, or suspect censor in this play,
but A STAR that guides your
co-spirit through And back again to
higher ground. This plateau is surmountable.

163.

⭐ Being aware of the daily world your children live in away from home is crucial. Try to KNOW their pals. The degree of pressure your kiddos feel is directly related to the petite country of friends that surrounds them. Keep a conversation going that is blessed by more listening than talking (sooo hard to do). Never forsake your tea parties: set everything out before them, even if they walk on by.

Take some road trips that insulate both of you. Pretend the

Radio is on the Fritz. Some of our best talks have happened in the car... where and when the routines that spin us to and fro have mercy. Click off all else and click on mother and child.

Make a gigantic effort to remember how you felt as a teenager, then fast-forward the trauma into this moment of pop culture: For this GENERATION, it is simply much harder, riskier, and graver

165.

this time around. And these extreme

circumstances require extreme

U I G I L A N C E.

I'm sure you've seen

and heard the ads for crisis

centers: "If you don't get help

from ... please get help from

OUR CENTER

somewhere. As the posted list of symptoms

flashes across the screen, do some folks

you know come to mind as potential

candidates... yourself included?

Filter the semi-NORMAL growing pains from
the ominous ROAD blocks that MAY
threaten THE HEALthy
child you love sooooo much.

Continue to Read and participate
within your world close at hand
and on a national level. No one
today, especially a mother, can
afford a vacation from responsibility.
While you have been
guarding your young, the rest of

167.

the commercial world has been hard
at work cultivating a VASt Plowed
field of future cash. ☆(It is truly
Amazing that many of these TILLERs
of GREED are parents themselves.)
So watch what kiddos read...see
what they see, and hear what they hear...to
help them digest this cultural
Buffet. Obsessively thin bodies,
material consumption to the point
that we are what we <u>own</u>, and

A high disregard for deferred gratification and life itself may rock your steady boat toward capsizing. Right this minute DONNA Reed is probably in heaven's eternal therapy program, along with Beaver's mother, June. Lord knows the rest of us are interested in a nice easy plan, right here, right now!! Oh, such tough puzzles a mother must study! Mercy!

today
celestial support group
10AM

MERCY

169.

Invest in the innate good of your child's soul, forgive mistakes, forget words hurled in RASH ANGER, let go of what you don't understand. A comprehension that is reasonable may not be possible at this time. If ever. You ARE A BRAVE mother on patrol: MARCH TALL. And try so very hard to measure every word, facial expression, and tone that may begin A WAR that Gandhi couldn't begin to fix....xoxo. Sometimes it's A kinder peace that comes when you choose to be fair and happy instead of always RIGHT.

Hold ON tight

170.

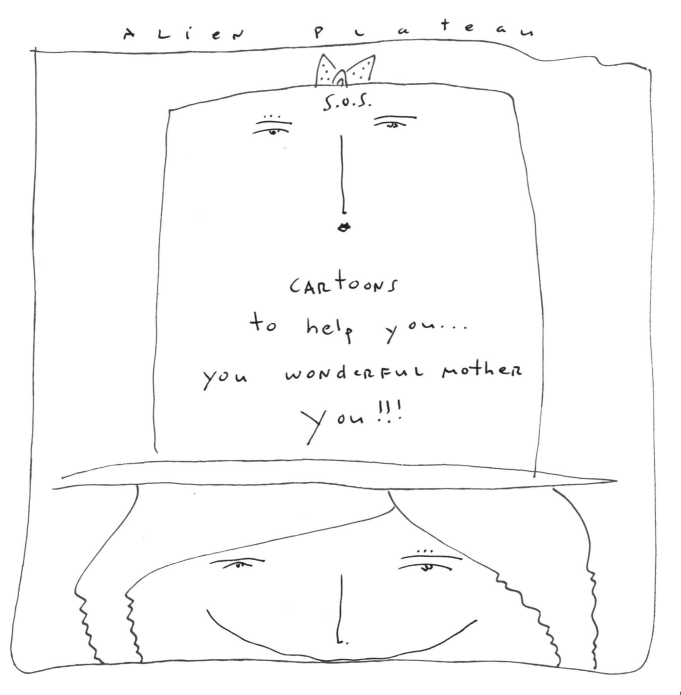

171.

To the Furthest Horizons....

SEND
ALL your Guilt
AWAY....

It is very, very toxic for

you...

And, ya know what, dolly???
you do not DESERVE it.

172.

ENGAGING A STELLAR MALE
ROLE MODEL FOR
★
YOUR
YOUNG
is peace of Mind and Heart
in
A
MOTHER'S BANK.

grand
dAd

dAd

PAL

uncle

A good-Egg-guy

173.

HAve

A Bevy of GiRl FRiends on

StAnd-By to help you

LeA ven

your deepest FeaRs And

w o R R i e s...

A Bevy need only be

A good stRong Few.

174.

TAME AND
COMBAT
HUMAN RAGE
with

A HEART AS BIG AS ALASKA
A MIND AS CALM AS FAIRY
Dust
A SOUL AS MASTERFUL AS AN
OLYMPIAN
STAR.

175.

DEAR CONGRESSMAN _____:

Please consider my thoughts

AS A citizen AND Mother....

thank
you...

Signed: _____ Date _____

Remember:

A teenager is a robin testing a soon-to-be flight plan.. Prepare for jolts and bumps before the big "send-off."

Webster's: MAture (adj.) ① Full-grown, ripe ② fully developed, perfected, etc.

It's the "etc."...and all that comes before... that takes a lifetime.

The making of Healthy Future Bosses...

Who shall be the Boss of Life itself? Let trusty Forces of Wisdom and Patient Study guide each day of your mothering toward a Higher than High Mountaintop of divine grace and Fulfilled Purpose.

Part-time Angels collect Nifty benefits eventually, dolly.

CHAPTER VII.

G.Q.

W.

Nice suits... oxfords

Stylishly pressed...

FAUX GROWN-UPS (in their late teens and beyond)

Handsome... pretty little elves of youth hidden inside adult-like frames... Do Not be Fooled, sweet good Mothers, your career is reaching it's peak!!! Retirement is For postal workers And Amway pioneers. Breathe deeply!!! And do carry on.

Only MOM can love And LEAD beyond compare... mon cheri.

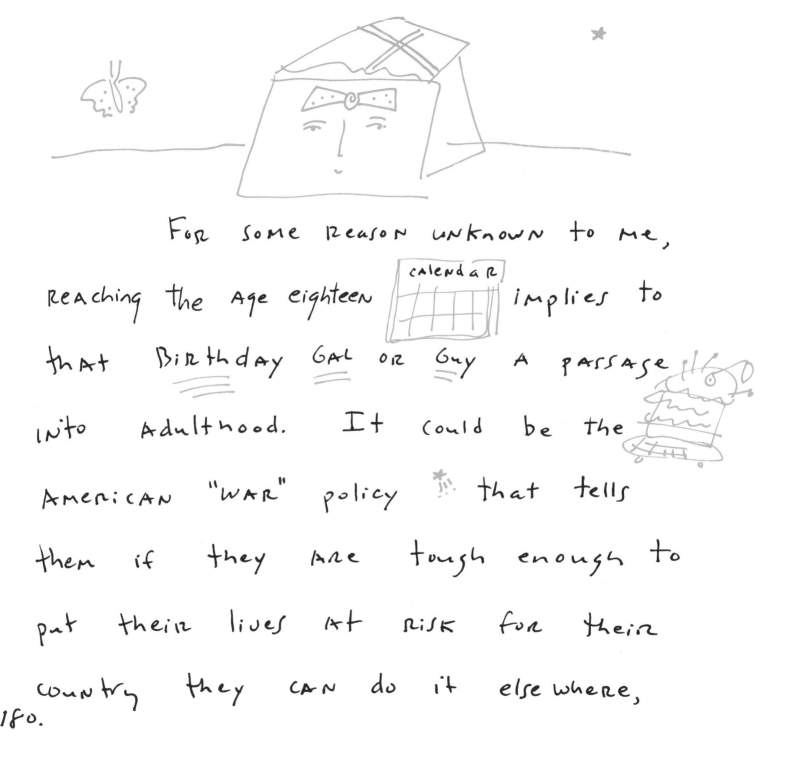

For some reason unknown to me, reaching the age eighteen [calendar] implies to that Birthday Gal or Guy a passage into adulthood. It could be the American "War" policy that tells them if they are tough enough to put their lives at risk for their country they can do it elsewhere, too.

without the buzz cut and uniform.
Actually the "Fields of College" can
be just as daunting as a call
for duty overseas, a patrolling for
peace in the midst of foreign faces.
The difference on a campus is that
they SELF-PATROL ON A MISSION OF Discovery
where Pinocchio Land mines luringly
await them in the company of other young
strangers assigned to the same mission.

181

Some casualties are inevitable.

So what is a mother to do when the real world is a semi-war zone... and college is your child's next tour?? The kiddo may <u>look</u> together in a nice Gap ensemble or tattered Goodwill ensemble, and will definitely attest to his or her readiness to fly, but how will

you know if they are indeed
ready to live independent of ☆...
your cautionary guard? Well,
there is no way to know ... NONE,
★ and that is the inside-out
truth. Remember the feeling you
loved as a small passenger in
the backseat of your father's
car when he would, for fun,
at your pleading, speed up over

183.

bumps or little hills... A [face drawing] weeee!

fleeting rush, both chilling and
delightful, danced upon your heart's
center stage.
That very sensation does an encore
for a mother who little by Big watches

her young GO. No car or hill necessary.

So you see 👓, those earlier
pages in your book when your nerves
flip-flopped over the first bike ride, turn
at bat with two outs, strike solo
performance in a play star at

184.

school,   swimming in the deep
                              (bigger than a Lego)
end,   driving a car ... All collide

as test runs for that day you

empty their boxed possessions into
                  (this big ☐)
A dorm room,   walk down the side-

walk, and drive away.   Waving "so

long" through the window will be A mega-

kleenex moment... you won't soon

forget.   jeepers...weepers

Many mothers pray, cross

185.

their fingers, visualize positive thoughts recite rosaries, and basically twitch through that "college" passage.

My first time, with Mitt... was pretty fair. As the weeks passed and I could not see what he was doing, a blind was lowered over my worry zone. And the phone calls were nice... surely up and down... but nice!!!

186.

You know...

The regular roommate trouble... bad food, ACADEMY AWARD whining over how terribly hard it all was. I did notice then, when I called him, he was often out (at the basketball courts or most probably at a party...) His astute roommate was good, however, at saying he was at the library... "exhausted, Mrs. Drew."

My second child gave us many curveballs. One of the most

187.

curving and disturbing was going off to college And in short time... Returning home. This child was not ready. And so with battle wounds and scars that remain in her youthful registry and in my own motherly repertoire, we climbed a few mountains that made the Rockies Look like Pancakes.

There is a velcro theory

in parenting... that if you are equipped with the velcro on one teaching hand and try to affix your lessons to a student's hand that has not yet discovered Velcro... you and those lessons remain unstuck.

This Velcro is not offered in a catalog, and comes in two styles: innate and earned, the latter coming from life experiences that may offer surprises requiring Divine CPR.

Thus far Anna, the second time around, has earned her B.F.A. with

HONORS!! She is her very own Artist, with a clear, true Voice. The best report card of all is the one that says her heart's mind and soul's spirit are on THE REAL HONOR ROLL. There should be a bumper sticker for parents with children on THIS... OH - SO - IMPORTANT LIST.

P ~~R O U~~ D ??? grateful

I am the exhausted upside-down parent whose child fell down a ^range of ^mountains and climbed ^back ^to the PEAKS... where I PRAY she has taken up permanent residence...

HALLELUJAH

Before this Faux Grown-up chapter in their lives, you have no doubt tried with all your "mother" HEART to give them the "tools" (invisible gifts) for their Toolbox. Unlike when you packed a Sack lunch or a duffle bag for camp, there is no sure checklist for you to evaluate. I think you have to shut your eyes and pray... "Dear God or _____, please give my child whatever else they need

that I may have missed. I love them
so and I know you do, too. When they
are away, and out of my sight... shadow
their follies and bring them back
home to me... oh please bring them
back home to me."

Never
ever
utter "Good Bye"...
whisper
"So long... Darlin,
I love you!"

teach
t h e m
the value of morality
and
the
inevitability
of
mortality...
in doses that are kind and
swallowably
Hopeful.

193.

THE
sweet magic
OF
Mother - in - lawing
And
GRANDMOTHERING

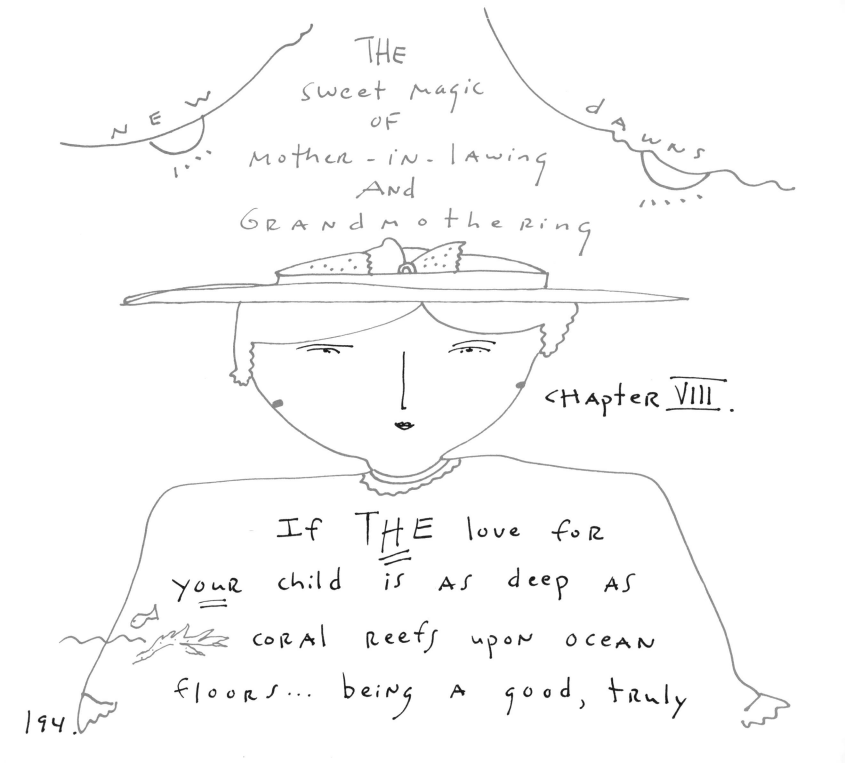

NEW dawns

CHAPTER VIII.

If THE love for your child is as deep as coral reefs upon ocean floors... being a good, truly good IN-LAW (second mom) and grand-mère is

possible.   Forget   the   corny   anecdotes

about   those   bitter   chatterboxes

that   live   ensconced   by   dreams

Never   lit.   They

Are   sad   and   exist   (thank good-

ness)   on   a   lonely   island

called   Minority.

I   Am   not   saying   it

195.

will be a three-layer chocolate cake picnic. There might be rich temptations to join those crabby apples on Minority Island. But this is your Bonus-Lotto to mother once again... deftly from the balcony upon velvet seats of sage.

Follow the lessons of remarkable women I have known,

196.

All heroes like the strongly rooted
souls of women before us, who
teach LESSONS IN LOVING WELL. And,
as for the power you hold within
your FAMILY, Remember this:
that very power of Mother-in-
Lawing can build dREAMS OR
destroy them... YOURS included.
THink
before you rule,
And MEASURE All words!

Sterling Mother-in-Law

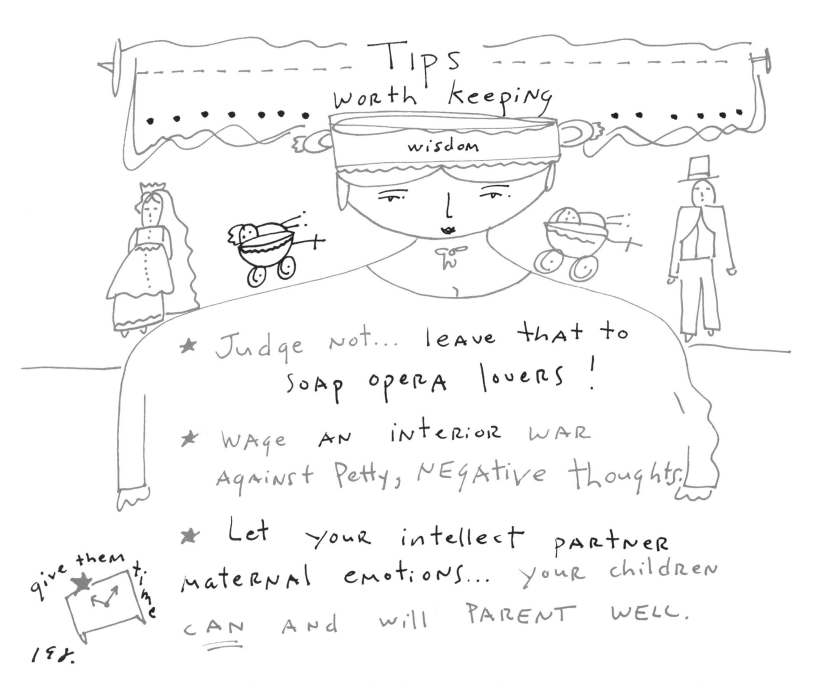

Tips worth keeping

wisdom

★ Judge not... leave that to soap opera lovers!

★ Wage an interior war against petty, negative thoughts.

★ Let your intellect partner maternal emotions... your children can and will PARENT WELL.

give them time

188.

★ Offer your best knowledge AS A buffet of truth that they can take or leave with your gracious blessing.

★ Let go of small hurts AND nagging details that pull you back to crossRoads of disappointment. This is a time FoR fresh chapters penned in platinum upon lily white hearts.

199.

★   Listen better than ever before with Buttoned Lips that only open upon invitation, un<u>less</u> your stewarding Heart sends a <u>clear</u> S.o.S. to unbutton them, dolly. CLEAR!! <u> </u>

    no selfish-static allowed!

★   Know that what your child sees in their chosen mate matters <u>more</u> than what you perhaps have <u>yet</u> to   see.

Mother-in-Lawing...

Decide

Well before they meet at altar's gate or selecting your coordinated beaded ensemble,

to

Let go of your own expectations and welcome

THEiRS.

I now pronounce you a DARN Good Mother-in-Law !!!

BRAVO!!

201.

GRANdmotheRing is the VERy, VERy best... so I'm told!

MY VERY own gRANdmotheRs gAve me A most tReAsuRed gift in the hours And days they loved me. I felt extra-ordinary And capable, bright, And Full of SUBSTANCE, because of the light within them thAt, As

luck had it, shone upon me!
Perhaps it is that simple...
We each have, step by step
the opportunity , to light
the way for one another, beaming
from interior lighthouses of
purpose tested by stormy spells
And comforted by joyful picnics,
As weather permits.
         If "spoiling" is a grand -

203.

motherly right, may you spoil
your little angels well.

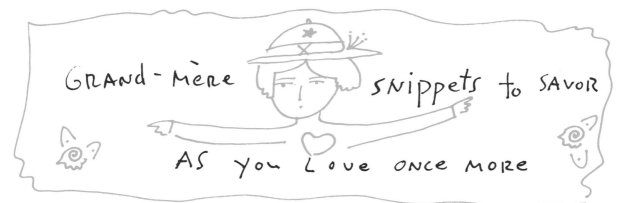

GRAND-Mère   snippets to savor

As you love once more

★ A part of this child is a
part of you. The rest is a
divine blend of what came
before. The landlord of this wondrous spirit resides elsewhere! As
a grandmother... resist all

temptation to possess, and
embrace what is shared in
the present moments of a
relationship that provides
unconditional love... This love
will give wings to your
beloved grandchild and a new
passport to your seasoned
mother's heart.
★   Give them silver change and

205.

copper pennies in a velvet pouch or shiny new wallet to spend in toy stores.

★ Splurge on Art supplies, keep a bounty of them on hand. Remember simple things to do from your childhood and teach and play again.

★ Baby-sit out of love, never out of martyrdom or a false

wish to revisit parenting and erase mistakes with a new model.

★ Cook and bake together: old dishes, family recipes that gave you a sense of warmth and place as you traveled to grown-up land.

MEAT + Rice Stew

★ Make scrapbooks and photo-memory books together. Two copies.

★ As these little ones grow, plan mini-trips (even if only for a day) that are exclusively for that child. Incorporate a wee bit of MODERN Fun with something else... like a museum stroll, nature discovery, or train ride to the Town next door.

★ Build a library of classic books to be read aloud and kept FOREVER.

Pen the name of each child, the date of gifting, and a little message of love from you... so that as they read these tales to their very own dollies one day, your heart will be felt as it wraps around each turning page.

★ Create a parade of tea parties. They are magical retreats, full of

209.

surprises that come when you
stop the clock and mix sweets with
an imagination that is safely
given permission to play in
your loving presence.
✱ And finally, remember that
as you proudly present the color
photos to all... let the names of
your own children ring a glorious
compliment First: " And you must

see my Anna and Brian's Lilly in
this trick-or-treat outfit..."
As a mother you will want to
embrace both your own child AND
the grandchild that takes your
heart to the moon and back.

such a fine, fine   grand-mère you
                                              are.

211.

DOLL-FACE... xox

AND so you will Remain first
FoRever A mother. AND Lo AND behold
Look, A new glorious cloak is bestowed... AND
GRANdmotheRS
ARE moms with ♡ Ph.D's !!!

A

degRee well earned
ANd Applauded by
the clear-eyed, sweet
lambs you've shepherded
so well, with A deep
love, SApphire blue... it's!!
true!!

ON eARth ANd elsewhere,
There aRe many beginnings... many
good ANd fine beginnings
... perhaps with FEW middles but never
212.   ever   fiNAL ends.

GRAND-mère...

A Super-dooper satellite of
loving wisdom and tested talents,
ready for more moonbeams.

213.

GRANNY complex... CAN't stand the stocking cap image, so you want to be NAMed

Do-Dough or NANAW or anything that does not announce this CHAnge... PLeeez!! xox

GET -over- it.....

xox

you're a spring chicken with a brand new Flock... that's all.

214.

Mighty Fine Grandmothers

CAN be Trusty FLASHLIGHTS

when their own children are a

bit in the dark about theee

grandchildren..

☆

Just FLip the "on" switch

and WHOA.... Remarkable!!!

215.

ONE GRANDMOTHER TO ANOTHER AT THE

GROCERY...

the one on the left:

YA KNOW, I WAS listening to SANdy
the other dAy ANd she sounded
So together ANd smart... telling
the kids things I used to say

BY
Gosh... By Golly...

She Really WAS listening ANd
I hAd No idea!!!

the one on the Right:

Speechless

216.

Chapter IX.

So mysterious... the other TENtAcles of Mothering

When I was a teen-ager, in padded bra and frosted lipstick, I joined the non-organized fraternity of kids that did not like their mothers... At all. Now that my travels have taken me well beyond that side of the fence, I see the magic of a

different kind of mothering.
Not a bit like the aproned
Loretta Young, but the kind of
mothering that is found in
loving relatives, pals, and even
strangers. Just when, for
whatever reason, the mother—
child love boat hits rough waters...
a new life raft of Mothering
arrives!!! Think back, and I

*

218.

Know that in the happy
clouds of your memory,
even this very day, there
Are remarkable people who
have mothered you well.

This magic is part of a
wonderful backup plan for
All of us. It is a plan that,
no doubt, includes you, too,
As a participant. Look at

219.

these [quilt sketch] Quilts. One you
own, and others you just might
embellish in this Lifetime!

Quilt I: Yours!

A mother's love
and life nurture as
best one can... Often
there are jeweled patch/es
embroidered by
others, that
cousin   add Final tribute.   grand-
Iris   mère
                                          Rose
         Aunt Mary Ann
                              Mrs. Rigby
Mary   Susan

220.

Quilt II: Your Parents!!

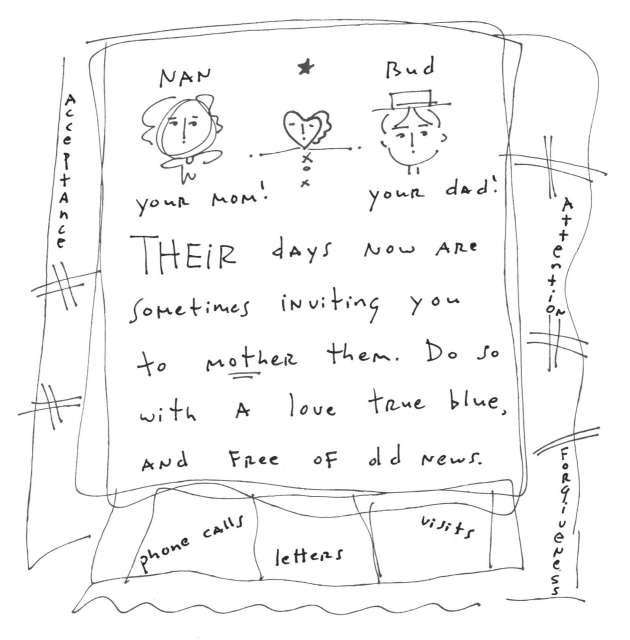

Quilt III : Aunt... or best pal or cousin or grand-mère... even volunteer!!

You, _____, can offer a dose of mothering every day to those who need it most. P.S. Remember, dolly, that sometimes it's A-O-K to mother your sweet SELF!!!

222.

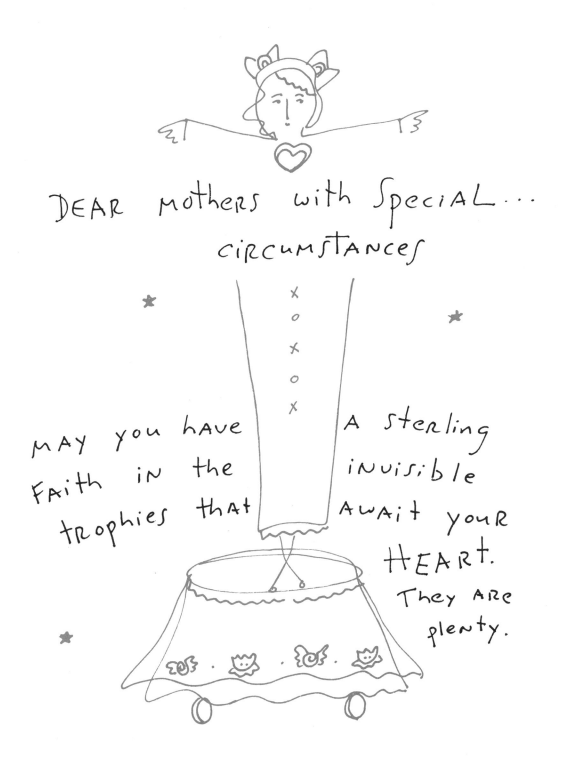

DEAR mothers with SpeciAL...
circumstances

MAY you have
FAith in the
trophies that

A sterling
invisible
AWAit your
HEART.
They ARE
plenty.

223.

An Adoptive Mother's Prayer...

Please, All heavenly mothers Above...
guide my heart steadfastly
toward this little heart I love
so deeply. Help me to create
a bond of truth and devotion,
unlike all others. One that
fits and stands on its very
own, even in patches of foggy
weather, and winds of doubt.
Blanket my mothering heart.

AMEN.

A Foster Mother's Prayer

Dear keepers of fragile hearts, keep my temporary watch* loving and deep. Let my spirit mother any wounds to a healing ground, where the promise of better days can be seen and touched. Thank you for the time I do have to gift wrap the heart of a child... for the journey before them.   Amen.

225.

A PRAYER

FOR mothers of children
that swim in troubled
waters...

Dear motherly guardians above,
please give me the strength to
carry on, without always fighting
to understand. Let my heart
continue to beat even though it is
breaking. Show me the way to
find the right help we need...
keep my mind sharp enough to
know the difference. Sit beside
my woes at night and give me a
wee bit respite. Amen.

Out of EARTHLY Sight

... Not touch

Children Are FRAgile MiRAcles
ON loAN. IN loss, Not dReAmt
oR WANted, PLEASE, God, help us.
Aunt PeARl sAys, "Loss cAN often
be A trAnslucent gAiN of soRts,
this odd MoNstRous trodding of
FAte,
giviNg us New unexpected visioNs
of pRomise". OH My, how Rich ouR heart's
trove, Ruby stitches felted iN FoReveR
Love knots.

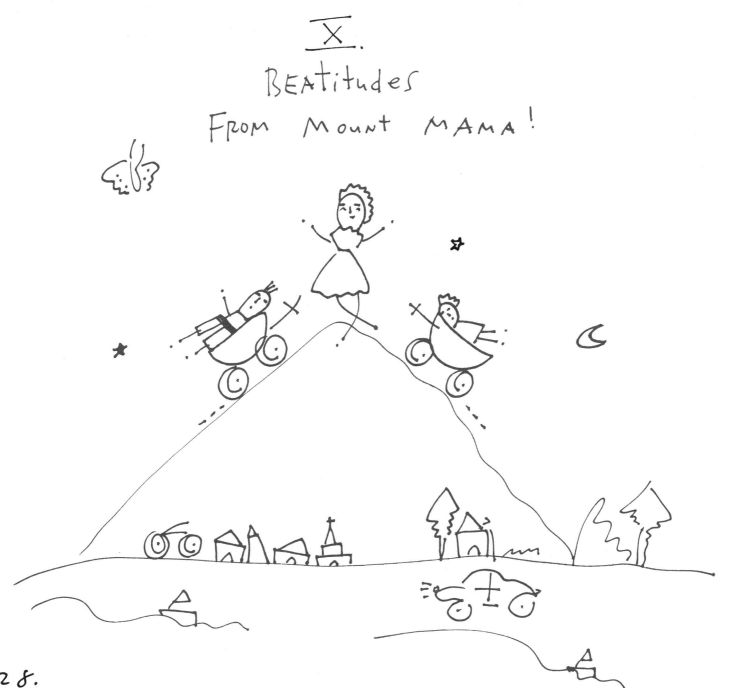

BEATITUDES
FOR Mothering
WELL

I. Bless those dear mothers who possess the Art of listening to small talk And BiG !!!

II. Blessed ARE All moms who every now And then... Allow themselves A darn good cry!! BRAVO!

III. Blessed ARE the WEARY moms who master the Art of RELAXATION!

IV. Blessed are those wonderfully fun moms who know how to play with their little ones... never too busy, either!

V. Blessed are the moms who do not cave in to bad daytime television, but carefully choose only the best!

VI. Blessed are those mothers who always know the intrinsic goodness of their child... no matter how naughty!

VII. Blessed are the Accepting mothers of what gold, silver, copper, or rusty tin may come their way. ✦

VIII. Blessed are the FLuiD, NIAGARA FALLS kind of moms, whose hearts find their way, ALWAYS, to the RIGHt SEA.

IX. Blessed are those MOMS who TEACH AND LEARN At the SAME time... remembering that All Report

CARDS VARY,

AND CAN be improved upon over time.

X. Blessed Are the wide-Awake Moms who Never, ever forsake their MATERNAL Antenna for All the Free And Pricey Advice in the world, whether given by theRApists, well-meaning family, Doctors, priests, or specialists of Any kind! Because their Doctorate in mothering Rules!!

Conclusion

THANK you foR Reading my book!! As A mother, I know how busy you ARe, And will AlwAys be. Even before life's pace quickened And TV dinners And FAX mAchines came Along... A mother's ♡ HeARt wAs the BusiEsT depot of energy on the face of this eARth. Nothing will change thAt. Not even A CAlgon bAth. You, dolly, ARe GRAND CENTRAl!

233.

For good mothering, whether in flesh or in spirit, keep these four things in mind : ✦

I. TAlent... you have more than you yet realize.

II. Courage... keep a wellspring of hard-work ethics and persistence that is HUGE.

III. Luck... your backyard, darlin, is full of four-leaf clovers.

✦ IV
And remember this... A good night's sleep is a great eraser.
Love
Nancy

234.